PRINCIPLES OF PRIMARY WOUND MANAGEMENT

A Guide to the Fundamentals
SECOND EDITION

Michael D. Mortiere, PA-C
Chief Physician Assistant
Department of Emergency Medicine
INOVA Alexandria Hospital
Alexandria, Virginia

Assistant Clinical Professor of Health Care Sciences
Department of Health Care Sciences
The George Washington University Medical Center
School of Medicine and Health Sciences
Washington, DC

D1062993

DEDICATION

To my wife, Diane, and my children, Meredith, Caroline, Patrick, and Kevin. Without their love, patience, cooperation, and understanding this book would not have been completed.

◆◆◆◆◆◆

NOTICE: Every effort has been made to assure that the indications and dosages of all drugs discussed in this book conform to the practices of the general medical community and have been recommended in the medical literature. From time to time, though, there may be changes in dosages, adverse reactions and indications. Therefore, it is recommended that a periodic review of the product inserts be made for updates approved by the FDA.

Coated vicryl, vicryl *RAPIDE*, PDS, monocryl, DERMABOND, and prolene are registered trademarks of Ethicon, Inc.
Augmentin is a registered trademark of SmithKline Beecham Pharmaceuticals.
Gelfoam is a registered trademark of Pharmacia & Upjohn.
Telfa is a registered trademark of The Kendall Company.
Adaptic is a registered trademark of Johnson & Johnson.
Xeroform is a registered trademark of Sherwood Davis+Geck.
ShurClens is a registered trademark of Convatec – A Bristol Myers Squibb Company.
AirStirrup is a registered trademark of Aircast, Inc.
Benadryl is a registered trademark of Pfizer.
ZeroWet Splashield is a registered trademark of Zerowet, Inc.
Irrijet is a registered trademark of Ackrad Laboratories, Inc.
RabAvert is a registered trademark of Chiron Corporation
Imovax is a registered trademark of Aventis Pasteur Inc.

Publisher: CLIFTON PUBLISHING
6109 Fox Run
Fairfax, Virginia 22030-5949 USA
(703) 502-3994   FAX (703) 502-1878
Internet: www.cliftonpublishing.com

Printer: United Graphics, Inc.
2916 Marshall Avenue
PO Box 559
Mattoon, IL 61938
217-235-7161   Fax 217-234-6274

CONTENTS

PREFACE

This text was written to offer all healthcare providers including, medical students, resident and attending physicians, physician assistants, nurse practitioners, and wound care specialists, a systematic and practical approach to primary wound care in the emergency department, clinic, office, field setting. All too often primary wound care is not adequately addressed in today's medical schools and allied health programs curricula despite the ever-increasing expectations by patients for excellence in health and wound care.

The second edition of *Principles of Primary Wound Management,* presents an orderly outline of the fundamentals; from the assessment of open and closed wounds to their repair. Like the first edition, it is formatted in this compact, pocket version the healthcare practitioner has rapid access to information on anatomy, local anesthetics, nerve block techniques, and advanced wound closure concerns. The orthopedic splinting section, with its illustrations, will make the proper selection and application of such devices easier. The text also touches upon some frequently asked questions and controversial topics in wound care.

This is not an exhaustive, all-inclusive text on wound care. The book does not discuss topics such as snake or insect bites and stings or describe procedures such as Z-plasty, replantation techniques, tendon repair, or nerve repair. It does however provide invaluable information to all who are faced with the daily demands of providing quality wound care. This book will most assuredly allow every practitioner to either develop or enhance their wound management skills and improve patient satisfaction.

SECTION 1

STERILE TECHNIQUE and INFECTION CONTROL

Before any health care provider initiates wound care, he/she must first be familiar with and put into practice the Universal Precautions guidelines established by the Centers for Disease Control (CDC). Likewise, one should always refer to their institution's policy regarding precautions for health care providers exposed to blood and other body fluids.

Many primary care providers forget that the operating room is *not* the only place for sterile technique. Although one does not have to scrub and don a surgical gown for every laceration repair, it is imperative that some simple measures be taken in the office, emergency department or clinic setting. At best, the suture room is clean - not sterile.

The following recommendations are offered to reduce the risk of contamination during any wound care procedure and are designed to help assure the maintenance of sterile technique:

1) Hands should be washed between patients and before all procedures.
2) Wear unsterile or sterile gloves when examining the wound for repair. Sterile gloves should always be worn when using sterile instruments or a sterile tray. Change sterile gloves between wound preparation and suturing procedures.
3) A surgical mask should be worn to prevent aerosol (droplet) contamination. This is a two-way street; aerosolization of saliva from the provider can contaminate the wound just as aerosolized blood and irrigation fluid can contact the provider.
4) Eye protection, whether prescription or clear lenses or face shields, must be worn to prevent droplet contamination into the provider's eyes.
5) The provider's hair, if long, should be contained with either a surgical cap or tie-back.
6) A laboratory coat or jacket should be removed prior to wound preparation and repair. This will prevent dragging long sleeves across a sterile operating field drape or the sterile suture tray. Likewise, long shirt sleeves should be rolled up.
7) NEVER recap contaminated sharps (needles, scalpels, etc.).

Care should always be taken to ensure sterility of the wound field, prep tray and suture tray. As a rule, anything that overhangs the Mayo stand or table is to be considered unsterile and contaminated. Similarly, any portion of the sterile tray or wound drape that becomes wet or comes in contact with an unsterile area is itself contaminated. At that point the tray or drapes must be replaced. All contaminated wound preparation items such as sponges and 4x4 gauze should be discarded in a nearby trash bucket and should never be returned to the sterile field.

SECTION 2

WOUND HEALING

One of the most important characteristics of all living things is the ability to self-repair. With few exceptions, an organism's own physiological mechanisms assist wound healing without external manipulation of its biochemical or cellular processes. Therefore, with an understanding of the human body's wound healing processes, one can better treat an injury and allow those natural healing mechanisms to progress.

In general, all wounds heal in one of three fashions: by primary intention, by secondary intention, or by tertiary intention.

PRIMARY INTENTION is the most efficient method of wound healing; resulting in faster healing times and generally a more cosmetically appealing scar. This method is most often chosen when the wound is clean and not likely to become infected.

Wound edges are apposed with sutures, staples or tape within a short period of time following injury - usually within 8 hours. The only exception to this widely-accepted "8-hour rule" pertains to facial, scalp and neck wounds which may be safely closed up to 24 hours from the time of injury. Of course this presumes that there is no gross tissue contamination (e.g., organic material). If any wound is grossly contaminated, cannot be thoroughly cleansed, or has a high index of suspicion in terms of infection potential; the wound edges should not be apposed primarily. Instead, the wound should be allowed to heal by secondary intention or a delayed repair may be contemplated.

Once the age of the wound is determined: 1) local anesthesia is administered, 2) the wound is cleansed and irrigated, 3) any necessary debridement is performed, and 4) the wound edges are apposed.

SECONDARY INTENTION involves the formation and contraction of granulation tissue. The consequences of this method of healing are 1) a longer healing period, 2) increased risk of infection because the wound remains open longer, and 3) a more unattractive scar.

Some reasons for allowing wounds to heal by secondary intention are: 1) an old wound (greater than 8 hours from injury to repair in all anatomic areas except the face, scalp, and neck); 2) a heavily contaminated wound (containing greater than 10^5 organisms per gram of tissue), including facial and head wounds unless adequate debridement or wound margin excision and cleansing can be accomplished; 3) an open wound with a large tissue defect, such as a large skin avulsion; 4) abrasions; 5) penetrating wounds such as bites and stab wounds; and 6) any infected, open wound.

TERTIARY INTENTION wound healing occurs when an untidy, old or contaminated wound is not sutured for the first 4-6 days following injury. Wounds are only repaired during this 4-6 day post-injury window only if

NO signs of infection are present at the time of closure. For this reason, tertiary intention healing is also known as *delayed primary closure, or repair*. Treating wounds in this fashion results in a healing time faster than wounds required to heal by secondary intention. In addition, because there is surgical intervention the cosmetic result is generally better than that of the wound allowed to heal secondarily. The exact procedure for initiating and performing a delayed primary closure is discussed in Section 11.

PHASES OF WOUND HEALING

Although the mechanisms of wound healing have been described in *phases*, they are by no means distinct entities or processes. They are mutually dependent processes. Depending upon the chosen reference text, wound healing will be classified into several phases. Here we will discuss four phases of wound healing: *inflammation, epithelialization, collagen synthesis,* and *scar maturation*. Under ideal conditions the following over-simplified scheme of wound healing takes place.

INFLAMMATION is initiated by an injury to the tissues and is manifested by the leaking of various substrates (i.e., histamine, enzymes, other proteins, and blood cells) into the surrounding tissues. This results in localized edema. Polymorphonuclear (PMN) leukocytes begin the task of removing cellular debris, bacteria, and foreign materials.

EPITHELIALIZATION begins within 12 hours of tissue injury. During this time, epithelial cells begin to migrate from the wound margins to cover the defect; thus preventing bacteria and toxic agents from readily entering the wound. Most primarily repaired wounds are "sealed" or "bridged" with epithelial cells within 24-48 hours after repair. However, open wounds or those wounds allowed to heal without intervention, require a longer completion time for epithelialization. This longer time frame is due to the active contraction of the epithelial cells to achieve final wound closure.

COLLAGEN SYNTHESIS begins after the inflammatory phase has deposited the necessary substrates into the wound site. Fibroblast proliferation and the resulting secretion of collagen by the fibroblasts begins by about the fourth day post-injury and continues for approximately six weeks. The appearance of the wound edges is more erythematous and raised; thus the term "healing ridge" has been given to this area abundant with new collagen and capillary beds.

SCAR MATURATION starts approximately six weeks after injury. During this phase, collagen synthesis and breakdown are in equilibrium. The collagen (scar) becomes more highly structured through cross-linking and reorientation. At this time the skin has regained at least 50% of its original tensile strength. Over the next year or so, the scar will flatten, contract, and fade to a normal skin tone. The wound can now be considered healed.

FACTORS AFFECTING WOUND HEALING

Many factors can influence the wound healing processes, including infection: blood supply to tissues, the mechanism of injury, the time lapse from injury to definitive treatment, the type of tissue injured, the presence of a foreign body or hematoma, the surgical technique used to repair the wound, the age and general health of the patient. The scope of this discussion is not to go into every detail of these factors but instead to outline the issues that the health care provider can and cannot control.

Of all the factors adversely affecting wound healing, infection is the most common. In the presence of infection, all the phases of normal wound healing are interrupted and any new tissue becomes necrotic. Infections may result from hematoma formation in the wound, an abundance of necrotic tissue, foreign body retention, inadequate wound preparation, or poor post-operative care.

The presence of a hematoma in a wound serves as a nidus for infection by creating an excellent culture medium for bacterial growth. Additionally, normal tissue healing is retarded because the hematoma exerts undue tension on the wound edges; thus decreasing tissue oxygen tension.

Active arterial or venous bleeding must be recognized and controlled prior to closure. If the bleeding cannot be controlled with local pressure or a vasoconstrictor added to the local anesthetic, then the bleeder *may* need to be isolated and ligated or cauterized. *One should always be mindful not to ligate nerves, which are usually in close proximity to the blood vessels. Likewise, one should never clamp or ligate anything in a bloody field; particularly in the hand!* Defer arterial bleeders in the hand to a hand specialist.

Necrotic tissue should be debrided or excised whenever feasible to ensure more tidy wound edges and decrease the risk of infection. Foreign particles (wood, glass, plastic, grass, stones, etc.) retained in the wound decreases the threshold for infection. When a small foreign body is implanted or left in the tissue, it often becomes encapsulated by fibrous tissue. This can cause discomfort or a disfiguring lesion which would require subsequent excision.

A good blood supply to the injured wound edges is critical as it provides the necessary oxygen and nutrients to and removes waste products from the site of injury. Wounds in areas with a poorer blood supply heal slower than those areas with excellent perfusion. It has been demonstrated that persons with a chronic low hematocrit (<14%) heal slower due to decreased oxygen tension at the wound edge. An example of this would be the relative poorer perfusion of the pre-tibial surface compared to the superior blood supply of the face.

Not only must there be good perfusion to the injured site but there must also be adequate drainage from the wound. For example, a distally-based flap laceration to the same pre-tibial area has a poor chance of survival secondary to venous congestion and edema in the flap. When the leg is kept in a gravity-dependent position (below the heart), the flap easily receives the blood it needs but it cannot drain blood from the flap; thus leading to venous pooling, infection, and/or necrosis. This simple example does not take into account any underlying medical condition, such as diabetes or immunosuppression, that may further complicate the normal healing processes.

Chronic medical problems can also have an adverse effect upon wound healing. Severe anemia, protein deficiency and vitamin C deficiency have been implicated as causes of delayed wound healing. Severe protein deficiency results in decreased fibroblast proliferation and subsequent decreased collagen synthesis. Since ascorbic acid is essential for collagen synthesis, a severe deficiency in this vitamin will result in impaired wound healing. Therefore, assessment of the patient's general health at the time of the wound repair and stressing a reasonably balanced diet is important to maintain normal healing function.

Diabetic patients are at high risk for wound infection and poor healing due to peripheral microvascular disease. Diabetics with open wounds, especially to areas of relatively poor vascularity (i.e., any lower extremity wound), should be carefully followed-up by their regular health care provider. Particular attention must be given to extremity elevation, frequent dressing changes and wound cleansing, as well as appropriate measures to control blood glucose levels.

Persons receiving steroids orally or parenterally tend to develop very friable tissue. For this reason, gentle tissue manipulation and placement of as few sutures as possible is strongly advised. Exogenous corticosteroids given in the first three days after injury will inhibit wound healing by reducing the inflammatory and collagen synthesis phases of healing. Corticosteroids also affect wound contraction mechanisms of sutured and nonsutured wounds alike.

There is an abundance of anecdotal reports in popular consumer magazines and Internet references in support of the use of vitamin E, coca butter or other cosmecuetical moisturizers on wounds to reduce scar formation. Despite these testimonials, there is no scientific evidence supporting that the use of over-the-counter topical agents improves the cosmetic appearance of scars. In fact, one recent study concluded that there was a high incidence of contact dermatitis related to vitamin E usage and that its use should therefore be discouraged. (Baumann, LS, Spencer J, *Dermatologic Surgery 1999;*25 (4), 311-315).

HYPERTROPHIC SCARS AND KELOIDS

Keloids are large, firm masses of scar tissue that are characterized by their ability to extend beyond the original wound margins. Due to the excessive proliferation of collagen, the wound margins are never visible. Keloids usually occur on the arms, elbows, shoulders, ears, waist, and sternum. Patients of Mediterranean or Black heritage tend to be predisposed to keloid formation. Preventive measures, although not always successful, include pressure dressings, tension-free closures, grafts and irradiation of the scar tissue, and steroid injection into the scar. Excision and attempts to revise keloids almost always result in larger keloid formation.

Hypertrophic scars, unlike keloids, remain within the confines of the original wound. They may appear slightly raised or markedly elevated. Hypertrophic scars are believed to be caused by wound tension and therefore can be found mostly over areas of movement or tension. In contrast to the keloid, hypertrophic scars may become smaller in size as they mature.

WOUND ASSESSMENT and DOCUMENTATION

Wound assessment in the primary care or emergency department setting should always be conducted in a systematic fashion. It is important to remember that first appearances can be deceiving. Elicit the mechanism of injury and examine the whole patient instead of concentrating on one obvious wound or injury. All too often significant underlying or hidden injuries have been neglected or missed beneath clothing or hair. Always follow ACLS and ATLS guidelines *before* caring for any wound.

Many health care providers begin wound closure without obtaining a thorough history or completing the examination of the patient. Such practices may lead to missed injuries, improper treatment, potentially serious complications, and possible litigation.

Jewelry must be removed from around the injured site, especially rings, bracelets and watches on an affected extremity. Failure to do so may cause such objects to act as tourniquets; resulting in tissue ischemia obscure radiographic studies, or result in digit loss if the edema worsens.

Regardless of whether the health care provider uses a standard SOAP note format or a customized wound record form, the following information must be obtained during the examination and documented:

- The type of injury, such as a laceration, abrasion, burn, or bite.

- The mechanism of injury, such as knife, glass, blunt trauma or mouth.

- The time lapse from injury to repair.

- Any pre-hospital care, including cleansing with soap and water, bandages.

- Prior medical history, including tetanus immunization status, drug allergies, current medications, previous injury or impairment, and pregnancy and last known menstrual period.

- Was the injury work related?

- For patients with hand injuries:
    Is the patient right or left handed?
    Ascertain the exact position of the hand at the time of injury.

If following the SOAP note format, one should include the responses from the above questions under the Subjective (S), as demonstrated below:

S: "19 y.o male to the E.D. c/o laceration to the right middle finger on a broken beer bottle at work <30 minutes PTA. PMH: neg. No meds. No known drug allergies. Right hand dominant. Pt. cleaned hand with soap and water PTA. Hand was in flexed position at time of injury. No other injuries."

Once the preceding information is obtained, assessment of the neurological, motor, and vascular function as well as the physical description of the wound can begin. The patient should be supine and made as comfortable as possible. Description of the wound must include the following:

- The **LENGTH** of the wound, in centimeters. Measure it.

- The anatomical **LOCATION** of the wound. Be as precise as possible. Drawings are often useful.

- A description of the **WOUND EDGES** - tidy or untidy.

- The **DEPTH** of the wound (i.e., "partial-thickness", "full-thickness", "into muscle", or "to bone").

- A notation about the presence or absence of **FOREIGN BODIES**. This may not always be possible, unless there is gross contamination or until after the wound is prepped. Also note the removal of any foreign bodies.

- A notation about any **FRACTURES, TENDON INJURY, DISLOCATIONS, AND RADIOLOGICAL RESULTS.**

- An assessment of the **NEURO-MOTOR-VASCULAR** status at the wound site and distal to the wound site. This must be accomplished **prior to** the administration of any local infiltration or nerve block anesthesia and repair.

ASSESSMENT OF SENSORY FUNCTION

Evaluating skin sensibility, either grossly or quantitatively, is important prior to the administration of local anesthesia. In general, checking sensation to light and sharp touch is all that is needed. However, two-point discrimination (2 PD) is recommended for any patient with a hand or finger injury. This sensitive examination allows the health care provider to quantitatively assess sensation. This becomes a useful tool to objectively monitor the patient's sensory improvement or deterioration during follow-up visits.

Two-point Discrimination Values for Fingers

Normal	1-6 mm
Fair	7-10 mm
Poor	11-15 mm
Anesthetic =	no points perceived

To perform this examination one may use a paper clip, ECG calipers, or the points of iris scissors (Fig. 3.1). The two points are opened to about 6 millimeters. The patient is then told that the points will touch the skin at the tips of the fingers and there will not be pain. The patient is further instructed not to look at the finger during the test so as not to skew the results.

The points are then placed against the skin

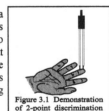

Figure 3.1 Demonstration of 2-point discrimination test with ECG calipers on the finger tip (see text).

first on one border and then the other border of the fingertip along the longitudinal axis. Light pressure is applied so as not to blanch the skin. Each time the patient is touched and perceives the points, he/she should be asked, "How many points do you feel." If the patient is able to perceive the two points at a distance 6 mm or less, sensation to that border of the finger is considered normal.

ASSESSMENT OF MOTOR FUNCTION

When assessing the motor function at the wound site, one should have an understanding of the underlying anatomy. For example, assume a patient presents with a transverse laceration to the volar surface of the middle finger just proximal to the proximal interphalangeal joint (PIPJ). The health care provider should not just ask the patient to make a fist and claim the tendon examination was satisfactory. Based upon that poor examination technique, the provider may have missed a partial laceration to either the flexor digitorum superficialis (FDS) or flexor digitorum profundus tendon (FDP), or both. Examination of the muscles and tendons of the hand will be discussed in detail in Section 5.

ASSESSMENT OF VASCULAR FUNCTION

Digital perfusion testing can be as simple as checking the capillary refill of the nail bed or noting the skin color to the injured area. It may involve the use of a doppler to assess blood flow through large vessels such as the popliteal or dorsalis pedis arteries. In most cases, however, simply palpating the distal pulses is sufficient.

When assessing the blood flow to the hand, one should routinely perform the Allen test. To perform this exam, exsanguinate the hand by elevation while the patient's hand is held in a fist. The provider then places his thumbs over the radial and ulnar arteries at the wrist. The patient is then asked to extend his fingers; but not fully. The palm should appear blanched or pale relative to the surrounding tissues. The provider will release the thumb over one of the arteries and observe the hand "pink up," within 2 - 5 seconds if the artery is patent and normal. The process is repeated for the other artery and the revascularization results documented.

All of the above information and examination results should be included in the Objective (O) portion of the SOAP note, as follows:

O: 1.5 cm tidy, transverse laceration to the volar surface of the right middle finger proximal to the PIPJ. Extends to tendon: FDS, FDP intact. Extension, abduction, adduction intact. Neuro: anesthetic, radial border. 2 PD ulnar border 5 mm. Digital artery bleed/lac noted radial border. No foreign bodies or fracture on exam.

The Assessment (A) portion of the SOAP note concisely states the nature of the injury. Using the previous example it might read:

A: Right middle finger laceration with digital nerve/artery laceration.

The Plan (P) section of the note should contain the following:

- The type of local anesthetic used, if any.
- The amount and route of administration of the local anesthetic agent, such as "via local infiltration", "MCP nerve block", "infraorbital nerve block", etc.
- The type of wound preparation performed, such as "betadine scrub, normal saline irrigation x 300 cc."
- Debridement, wound margin excision, undermining, or other procedures, when performed.
- Foreign body removal, when applicable.
- Wound repair, including type, size, and number of sutures for each tissue layer repaired.
- The type of wound dressing applied (i.e., Adaptic®, xeroform gauze, bulky dressing, type of splint).
- Disposition note, including follow-up care, suture removal / wound check instructions.

Using the same patient, the Plan (P) might read:

P: Anesthesia: 2% lidocaine plain 3 cc via MCP nerve block.
Betadine scrub, normal saline irrigation x 300 cc
5-0 nylon x 3 skin, xeroform and bulky dressing applied.
f/u: call hand surgeon in a.m. for earliest appointment.
keep hand elevated, clean and dry; return if signs of infection develop.
Take antibiotics as directed until none remain.

WOUND CLASSIFICATION

Soft tissue injuries are generally classified by their appearance and by the causative mechanism. It is important to differentiate between such wounds because the treatment for one type of wound may not fit the treatment plan of another. Never take any wound at face value. Instead, make every effort to ascertain the mechanism, the age of the wound, and into which classification scheme it falls.

For example, a wound may appear small, clean and incision-like on the exterior; leading one to believe it is just a superficial laceration. In actuality, the wound may extend deep into the subcutaneous tissues and may have had introduced into it clothing or other contaminants. Such a deep stab or puncture wound would usually not be closed primarily unless the full depth of the wound could be determined and the wound was thoroughly cleansed. Primary closure of such wounds would usually increase the likelihood of infection.

On the other hand, if a wound was made with a razor and the wound margins are long, its depth was easily determined to be full-thickness, and no contaminants were visible; it could have been repaired primarily.

LACERATIONS

By definition, a laceration is a wound resulting from the tearing or shredding of tissue by blunt forces. In contrast, an incision is a wound made by a sharp tool or instrument. Since most wounds seen in the emergency department or primary care setting are not planned, operating room-type incisions, clinicians refer to traumatic, incision-like wounds as **lacerations**.

Lacerations may be linear or stellate. They should be described as tidy or untidy. Tidy simply means the wound margins are cleanly cut or have little visible damage. Untidy lacerations may be jagged, abraded, contused, or grossly contaminated. The margins of the untidy laceration should be surgically debrided or excised, whenever possible, to remove necrotic tissue. Lacerations may result from contact with almost any object, including pieces of metal, glass, or blunt trauma.

ABRASIONS

Wounds in which the epidermis or dermis has been removed by friction are called **abrasions**. A well-known example of this type of wound is the common childhood injury - the scraped knee. However, abrasions can present more dramatically. An abrasion resulting from contact with the surface of pavement (also known as "road rashes" or "road burns") usually involves large areas of skin. Failure to thoroughly cleanse debris and debride all nonviable tissue may result in permanent traumatic "tatooing" of the skin from imbedded road particles. Furthermore, such road particles greatly decrease the threshold for infection; thus increasing the probability for a wound infection and an unappealing scar.

AVULSIONS

An **avulsion** is a loss of soft tissues; from dermis to muscle. Most avulsions however are confined to the dermal and subcutaneous fatty layers of the skin. Many avulsions seen in the emergency department or primary care setting are the result of motor vehicle collisions (MVCs) or food preparation accidents.

Avulsion injuries from MVCs often arise when the patient's face strikes the windshield or even the rear-view mirror. Fortunately, most are smaller avulsions unlike those seen before the mid-1960's; before the advent of plastic-laminated windshield glass. Food service workers frequently sustain injuries to their fingers and hands from the improper or unsafe use of knives, meat slicers, food processors, or blenders.

Incomplete avulsions, also known as flap lacerations, pose a different and sometimes difficult management problem. Flaps with proximally-based pedicles have little or no interruption to their vasculature; thus allowing them to heal well. Distally-based pedicles, on the other hand, have a disruption in the venous drainage from the flap. Under ideal circumstances, restoration of a venous network to drain the flap takes approximately two days from the time of injury. Healing time and complications are affected by the amount of tissue disruption or tissue crush component. Venous congestion and pooling results especially if the flap is located on an extremity or in an area of relatively poor vascularity. The ultimate adverse consequences are edema, infection, and necrosis of the flap. To help counter this problem, gentle tissue handling and maintaining elevation of the affected extremity are essential.

PUNCTURE WOUNDS

Puncture wounds may be caused by a variety of objects such as needles, glass, nails, splintered wood or metal, knives, or ice picks. Although controversial among some in the medical community, puncture or stab wounds are generally not closed primarily because contaminants (i.e., clothing, skin flora, organic material) most likely were "injected" into deeper tissues and retained. Instead, such wounds of uncertain depth are anesthetized, cleansed, irrigated, dressed, and allowed to heal by secondary intention. Some wounds, particularly if they are large, may be candidates for a delayed primary repair.

At some institutions, stab wounds are closed primarily - with or without surgical drains put into place. In these instances, the depth of the wounds are presumed to be determined by open exploration. "Blind" probing of a penetrating neck, chest, or abdominal wound with a cotton-tipped applicator, or the like, should be discouraged.

Antibiotic therapy should be initiated when the risk of wound infection in puncture or stab wounds is deemed high.

DEGLOVING INJURIES

Degloving injuries occur most often to the upper and lower extremities. These injuries are can be caused be various forms of machinery (i.e., washing machines, newspaper printing presses, steel stamping machines). Degloving injuries, because of the tearing and crushing forces involved, result in the loss of a substantial amount of skin, including fat, muscle, tendons, and / or bone. Because of the severity of the injury, an immediate hand, orthopedic, or plastic surgery consult should be obtained.

MAMMALIAN BITES

Human bites carry with them a high rate of infection; therefore, almost all human bite wounds should not be closed primarily. The exception to this statement is that most facial wounds should be thoroughly cleansed, debrided, and repaired primarily. This practice is particularly important where permanent disfigurement is likely if the wound is not sutured. Preservation and coverage of cartilage and bone with skin is always a prime concern.

If the wound age or level of tissue contamination of a facial or neck wound is questionable, a delayed primary repair may be considered after the threat of infection has diminished (usually 4-6 days post-injury). All devitalized tissue should be removed by means of a thorough wound prep and surgical wound debridement or wound margin excision. One should always be careful not to debride too much tissue and leave a larger defect. Antibiotics are necessary for all but the most superficial wounds. Infected human bites, especially those to the hand, need to be admitted to the hospital for intravenous antibiotic therapy, incision and drainage.

Eighty percent (80%) of **Cat bites** (not scratches) become infected compared to five percent (5%) of dog bites. This appears to be due to the fact that the cat's teeth are needle-like; thus, injecting oral bacteria deep into the wound and soft tissues. Such wound infections are usually rapid with cellulitis occurring within 24 hours. The predominant pathogen is *Pasteurella multocida*. Cat bites should be cleansed, dressed, and splinted (if they cross a joint on the hand or foot). The patient should be instructed to keep the extremity elevated above heart level. Close follow-up should also be provided. Oral antibiotics such as amoxicillin/clavulanate (Augmentin®) alone or penicillin with ceftriaxone or doxycycline are recommended. The rabies status of the animal must also be investigated and post–exposure rabies prophylaxis initiated when necessary.

Dog bites can be sutured primarily provided they are: 1) less than 8 hours old, 2) not deep puncture wounds, 3) not infected, and 4) copiously irrigated, debrided or excised of all devitalized tissue. Individualized treatment should be given to dog bite wounds to the hand. Large hand wounds that have significant exposure of subcutaneous tissue or vital structures may require loose approximation of the wound margins, while smaller bites or punctures should be left open to heal secondarily.

While the normal oral flora of the dog's mouth includes *Pasteurella multocida*, the infection rates for dog bites is about 5 percent. This may be due in part to the fact that dog bites result in the shredding and crushing of tissue rather than the creation of deep punctures as seen in cat bites. Despite the relative low infection potential of a properly cleansed, irrigated, and de-brided dog bite wound, antibiotics are customarily recommended for 3 - 7 days. Amoxicillin/clavulanate (Augmentin®) is recommended.

As with cat and other mammalian bite wounds, the patients must be instructed to elevate the injured extremity to reduce additional edema. The rabies status of the animal must also be investigated and post–exposure rabies prophylaxis initiated when necessary.

SECTION 5

BASIC HAND and HEAD ANATOMY REVIEW

The majority of lacerations and other traumatic wounds which present to most large community or inner city hospitals are located on the hands, scalp, and face. Some statistics place these figures at 75% or higher. Therefore, the next few pages present a short review of the basic anatomy of the hand and some facial structures. Hopefully this will allow the provider to render a better examination of these areas of the body. As always, a good anatomy textbook and the availability of expert consultants will make a more difficult examination easier.

THE HAND

Over the last two decades or so, many health care providers have used confusing or contradictory terminology when describing the structures and areas of the hand. Anatomists have long taught that the hand and the wrist have anterior and posterior surfaces as well as medial and lateral borders. The anatomists are of course correct from a strictly anatomical position.

However, around 1978 the American Society for Surgery of the Hand (ASSH) adopted and encouraged the use of a standard hand terminology in clinical practice. This terminology is used by most hand specialists in documentation and communication with colleagues about injuries affecting hand structures. The ASSH's recommendations are presented below.

The hand and digits can be described as having a palmar or volar surface and a dorsal surface. In addition, the hand and digits have an ulnar border and a radial border. The palm is divided into three areas: the thenar eminence, the hypothenar eminence, and the mid-palm area. The thenar eminence is the muscular area on the volar surface of the hand overlying the thumb metacarpal. The hypothenar eminence is that muscular area on the volar surface of the hand overlying the fifth, or little finger, metacarpal. The mid-palmar area lies between the thenar and hypothenar eminences (Fig. 5.1).

The digits are *named* and should not be designated by numbers. The digits are (from radial border to ulnar border): the thumb, the index finger, the middle finger, the ring finger, and the little or small finger (Figs. 5.1 and 5.2).

Each finger has the following joints: the metacarpophalangeal joint (MCPJ), the proximal interphalangeal joint (PIPJ), and the distal interphalangeal joint (DIPJ). The thumb, however, has only metacarpophalangeal joint (MCPJ) and an interphalangeal joint (IPJ).

The hand is innervated by three nerves: the radial, the median, and the ulnar nerves. Each nerves has a sensory component and a motor component. Although variations to the typical sensory distribution pattern of these nerves have been noted, the most common sensory pattern is illustrated in Figure 5.3.

One may easily assess the MOTOR function of the radial, median, and ulnar nerves by performing the following simple tests:

Ask the patient to extend the wrist .... Radial nerve
Ask the patient to touch the tips of
 the thumb and little finger, forming a circle .... Median nerve
Ask the patient to abduct and adduct fingers .... Ulnar nerve

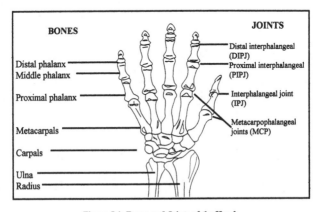

Figure 5.1 Bones and Joints of the Hand

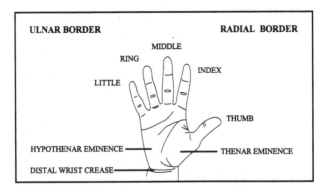

Figure 5.2 Surface anatomy of the hand (palmar view)

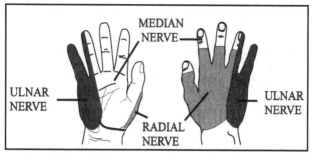

Figure 5.3 Typical sensory innervation pattern of the hand

Each digit has four digital nerve branches: 2 palmar branches and 2 dorsal branches. Nerve supply to the nailbed is derived from branches of the paired palmar digital nerves. The paired dorsal digital nerves provide sensation to the dorsal surfaces of the fingers from the MCP joint to just beyond the PIP joint (Fig. 5.4).

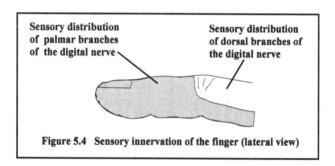

Figure 5.4 Sensory innervation of the finger (lateral view)

The muscles of the hand can be divided into two large groups: the **intrinsic** muscles and the **extrinsic** muscles. The extrinsic muscles of the hand have their origin in the forearm and their tendonous insertion in the hand while the intrinsics have both origin and insertion in the hand. The extrinsic group can be further subdivided into the extrinsic flexors and extrinsic extensor muscles. The extrinsic flexors are located on the volar surface of the hand and function to flex the digits and the wrist. The extrinsic extensors are located on the dorsal surface of the forearm and hand; they function to extend the digits and wrist.

As previously mentioned, muscle function should always be evaluated at and distal to the injury site. For injuries of the volar and dorsal surfaces of the hand and wrist, each muscle or group of muscles should be examined. Examination of the hand is clearly explained in Tables 5.1 a-c.

Table 5.1a   Intrinsic Muscles of the Hand and their Examination

Name of the Intrinsic Hand Muscles	How to Evaluate Muscle Function
THENAR GROUP (3 muscles)	
Abductor Pollicis Brevis (APB) Opponens Pollicis (OP) Flexor Pollicis Brevis (FPB)	Ask the patient to touch the tip of the thumb to the tip of the little finger or ask the patient to place the dorsum of the hand on the table and raise the thumb straight up (90° to palm).
HYPOTHENAR GROUP (3 muscles) Abductor Digiti Minimi (ADM) Flexor Digiti Minimi (FDM) Opponens Digiti Minimi (OPM)	Ask the patient to move the little finger in an ulnar direction while palpating the muscle mass and noting a dimpling of the skin.
Abductor Pollicis muscle (AdP)	Place a piece of paper between the thumb and the radial side of the index finger and attempt to pull it out. If the IPJ of the thumb flexes (Froment's sign), the muscle is weak or nonfunctioning. Check the opposite hand for comparison.
Interosseous muscles	The interossei insert onto the proximal phalanges of the fingers and abduct / adduct the fingers. The palmar interossei adduct while the dorsal interossei abduct the fingers away from and toward the middle finger.
Lumbrical muscles	Ask the patient to flex the MCPJs and extend the PIPJs and DIPJs of the fingers. Lumbricals are separate muscles that insert into the extensor mechanism.

Table 5.1b Extrinsic Flexor Muscles of the Hand and Wrist and their Examination

Name of Extrinsic Muscle	Tendon Insertion	How to Evaluate Tendon Function
FLEXORS		
Flexor Pollicis Longus (FPL)	Volar base of distal phalanx of the thumb	Ask the patient to bend the tip (IPJ) of the thumb.
Flexor Digitorum Profundus (FDP)	Volar base of distal phalanx of the index through little fingers	Ask the patient to bend the tip (DIP joint) of each finger while the examiner holds the PIPJ of that
Flexor Digitorum Superficialis (FDS)	Volar base of middle phalanx of the index through little fingers	Ask the patient to bend the PIPJ of each finger while the examiner holds the other fingers in extension (to block the FDP function).
Flexor Carpi Ulnaris (FCU)	Pisiform bone of the wrist	(
Flexor Carpi Radialis (FCR)	Volar aspect of the index metacarpal	(Ask the patient to flex the wrist while each of (these 3 tendons is palpated.
Palmaris Longus (PL)	Palmar fascia	((

Principles of Primary Wound Management

Table 5.1 c Extrinsic Extensor Muscles of the Hand and their Evaluation

Name of Extrinsic Muscle	Tendon Insertion	How to Evaluate Tendon Function
EXTENSORS		
Abductor Pollicis Longus (APL)	Dorsal base of thumb metacarpal	Ask the patient to bring the thumb out to the side of the hand while the examiner palpates each tendon over the radial border of the wrist.
Extensor Pollicis Brevis (EPB)	Dorsal base of proximal phalanx of the thumb	
Extensor Carpi Radialis Longus (ECRL)	Dorsal base of 2nd metacarpal	Ask the patient to make a fist and extend the wrist against resistance.
Extensor Carpi Radialis Brevis (ECRB)	Dorsal base of 3rd metacarpal	
Extensor Pollicis Longus (EPL)	Dorsal base of distal phalanx of the thumb	While placing the palm flat on the bed or table, ask
Extensor Digitorum Communis (EDC)	Dorsal base of middle and distal phalanges of each	Ask the patient to open or straighten out the fingers
Extensor Indicis Proprius (EIP)	Only on index finger. Ulnar to EDC.	Must be isolated from EDC by asking the patient to
Extensor Digiti Minimi (EDM)	Only on little finger.	Must be isolated from EDC by asking the patient to
Extensor Carpi Ulnaris (ECU)	Dorsal base of the little finger.	Palpate the tendon as the patient extends the wrist

NAILBED ANATOMY

Knowing the anatomy of the epionychium (Fig 5.5) is essential for the proper treatment of injuries to this region of the hand. The epionychium consists of the nail plate, the nail bed, and surrounding soft tissues.

The entire area beneath the nail plate is called the nail bed. The nail bed is comprised of the proximally-located germinal matrix and the distally-

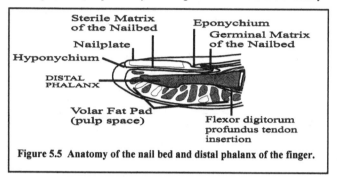

Figure 5.5 Anatomy of the nail bed and distal phalanx of the finger.

located sterile matrix. The germinal matrix extends beneath the proximal nail fold and represents the origin of the nail plate. Some also refer to this region as the "nail root". The sterile matrix is that portion of the nail plate distal to the lunula where the nail plate adheres to the nail bed.

The soft tissue proximal to the eponychium and overlying the proximal nail plate is the nail fold. The nail fold is divided into the (ventral) floor and the (dorsal) roof. The nail plate can be divided into the thin dorsal layer, the intermediate nail, and the ventral nail. The dorsal roof gives the thin surface of the nail its shiny appearance. The intermediate nail arises from the ventral floor of the nail fold proximal to the lunula. The intermediate nail represents a majority of the nail plate mass. The ventral nail plate extends from the lunula to the hyponychium. The ventral nail contributes to the thickness of the nail plate as it progresses from the lunula.

The paronychium is that tissue found on both sides of the nail plate. The hyponychium is the tissue found beneath the distal edge of the nail plate. The third area, which is the most proximal portion of the soft tissue in contact with the nail plate, is the eponychium. The lunula is the white crescent-shaped area of the nail plate just distal to the eponychium. Its appearance is due to the retention of keratohyalin and the nail plate not being completely cornified. The area beneath the lunula probably represents a point of non-adherence of the nail plate to the nail bed.

SCALP AND FACE

It would impossible to discuss every anatomical structure of the face and head in this text. Instead, only those structures which pose a particularly difficult wound management problem or are encountered frequently will be mentioned. One should always refer to an anatomy text to help illustrate pertinent anatomical structures and landmarks.

The galea aponeurosis is the dense connective tissue joining the frontalis and the occipitalis muscles. Other facial muscle groups are illustrated in Figure 5.6 below.

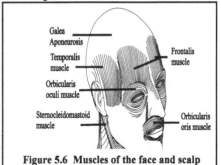

Figure 5.6 Muscles of the face and scalp

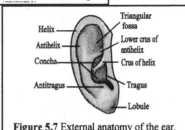

Figure 5.7 External anatomy of the ear.

Some important structures and landmarks around the mouth are: the orbicularis oris muscle, the philtrum and the vermilion cutaneous border of the lip (Fig. 5.8). The orbicularis oris muscle, which is circumferential to the oral cavity, is almost always injured following trauma to the mouth. The vermilion cutaneous border of

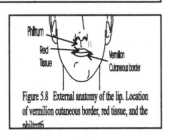

Figure 5.8 External anatomy of the lip. Location of vermilion cutaneous border, red tissue, and the philtrum.

the lip is the line that marks the junction of the red tissue of the lip and the surrounding skin of the upper or lower lips. Its accurate repair and avoidance of further tissue edge distortion during anesthetizing and repair of the wound is imperative.

An injury to the Facial nerve and/or the parotid (Stenson's) duct should always be ruled out when a patient sustains a laceration or puncture wound to the cheek. Large, repairable branches of the Facial nerve (buccal branches of cranial nerve VII) are between the stylomastoid foramen and a vertical line dropped from the lateral canthus of the ipsilateral eye. Branches medial to this imaginary vertical line are usually too fine to repair and will often regenerate satisfactorily (Fig. 5.9).

The parotid duct begins at the parotid gland and travels medially about midway along a line connecting the tragus of the ear and the mid-portion of the upper lip. At this midway point, the parotid duct orifice can be visualized on the buccal mucosa opposite the upper second bicuspid.

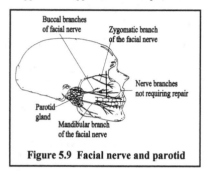

Figure 5.9 Facial nerve and parotid

DENTITION

Even though the scope of this text does not discuss the treatment of dental injuries, it is still imperative that one be able to correctly identify injured teeth. Figure 5.10 illustrates the surfaces for both deciduous and permanent teeth as well as the names and assigned numbers to make documentation easier. The labial surface refers to the front surface of the tooth that is adjacent to the cheek and lips. The lingual surface is the tooth surface toward the tongue.

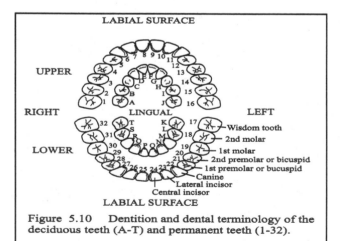

Figure 5.10   Dentition and dental terminology of the deciduous teeth (A-T) and permanent teeth (1-32).

LOCAL ANESTHETICS and ADMINISTRATION TECHNIQUES

The local anesthetic agents used today are divided into two classes: the esters and the amides. Although local anesthetics of the amide linkage group are used almost exclusively, some institutions may continue to use the ester-linked local anesthetic agents. The amides include lidocaine hydrochloride, bupivacaine hydrochloride, and mepivacaine hydrochloride. The most common ester-type local anesthetics include procaine hydrochloride and chloroprocaine hydrochloride.

Local anesthetics prevent both the conduction and generation of nerve impulses by preventing a large transient increase in the permeability of the nerve cell membrane to sodium ions. This progressively increases the threshold for electrical stimulation in the nerve; thus leading to a block in conduction. In general, the progression of anesthesia is related to the diameter, myelination, and conduction velocity of the affected nerve fibers. Pain is usually the first sensation to disappear, followed by temperature perception, touch, deep pressure, and finally loss of motor activity. The regression, or "wearing off", of the anesthesia occurs in the reverse order.

Ester-type local anesthetics are hydrolyzed by plasma cholinesterase to aminobenzoic acids and by esterases in the liver. Amide-type local anesthetics are metabolized primarily in the liver by microsomal enzymes. Because both classes of anesthetics are metabolized to some degree by the liver and excreted through the kidneys, patients with impaired hepatic or renal function risk developing toxic plasma concentrations of the drug or its metabolites. In addition, both types are excreted mainly in the urine as metabolites and as small amounts (5-10%) of the unchanged drug.

When using any local anesthetic, one should have resuscitation equipment and oxygen readily available. One should be familiar with the symptoms of allergic reactions, toxic reactions, and familial malignant hyperthermia.

Allergic reactions to the amide-type anesthetics have been linked to a preservative, methylparaben, in the multiple-dose vials. Methylparaben-free, single-dose vials are available for patients with such allergies. Most reactions, however, are the result of intravascular injection of the drug or an overdosage. Local reactions may manifest with pruritis or urticaria. Toxic reactions may be characterized by restlessness, anxiety, dizziness, blurred vision, tremors, slurred speech, or drowsiness. Symptoms may progress to seizures, respiratory depression, and cardiovascular collapse. It is extremely rare for cross-sensitivity between the ester and amide local anesthetics.

Table 6.1 compares and summarizes the solution concentrations, maximum doses, onset of action, and duration times of the most commonly used local anesthetics. For a more complete discussion of local anesthetics, please consult a pharmacology text or the product packaging insert. The onset and duration of any local anesthetic varies depending upon the type of

Table 6.1 Characteristics of Common Injectable Local Anesthetics

Generic Name (trade name)	Drug Class	Available Concentrations	Maximum Allowable Adult	Average Onset Time [2]	Average Duration Time [2]
Procaine (Novocain)	Ester	0.5%,1%, 2% solutions	1000 mg (10-15 mg/kg)	1 - 5 minutes	30 - 60 minutes
Lidocaine (Xylocaine)	Amide	0.5%,1%, 2% solutions	*without epi:* 300 mg (4.5 mg/kg) *with epi:* 500 mg	0.5 - 30 minutes; varies by route given	30 minutes to 3.5 hours
Mepivacaine (Carbocaine)	Amide	1%, 2% solutions	400 mg (4.5 mg/kg)	1 - 10 minutes	1 - 3 hours
Bupivacaine [3] (Marcaine, Sensorcaine)	Amide	0.25%, 0.5% solutions	*without epi:* 175 mg *with epi:*	2 - 30 minutes	8 - 16 hours

[1]   Adult doses. Pediatric doses to be calculated according to mg/kg or mg/lb body weight for specific agent. Children 3 yrs + (1.5 - 2 mg/lb; max. 75-100 mg). Consult product packing information for latest dosing information.

[2]   Dependent upon solution concentration, route of administration, addition of epinephrine, and individual patient response.

[3]   Use not recommended in children under 12 years of age.

anesthetic used, the presence or absence of a vasoconstrictor in the solution, the concentration of the solution, the route of administration, the type of block used, and the overall health of the patient.

Local anesthetic doses can be calculated easily using the following information:

0.5% solution =   5 mg of anesthetic per milliliter
1% solution   = 10 mg of anesthetic per milliliter
2% solution   = 20 mg of anesthetic per milliliter

Therefore, 20 ml of 1% lidocaine contains 200 mg of lidocaine hydrochloride.

The addition of a vasoconstrictor, such as **epinephrine,** to some anesthetic solutions decreases the rate at which the anesthetic is absorbed; thereby prolonging the duration of the anesthesia. Vasoconstrictors also decrease the systemic toxicity to the local anesthetic. When a local anesthetic with epinephrine is infiltrated into the tissues, a decrease in bleeding around the site is noted. This hemostatic action takes about 10 minutes to occur.

Even though anesthetics containing epinephrine are useful for hemostasis, they do have their limitations. Such agents should not be administered in the digits, the tip of the nose, the penis, and any area with end-arteries or poor collateral circulation. Vascular spasm, ischemia, or necrosis of the tissue at and distal to the injection site is therefore a legitimate concern.

Care should be exercised when considering the use of vasoconstrictors in areas, except the face, on patients with ischemic vascular disease or diabetes mellitus. Patients taking monoamine oxidase inhibitors, tricyclic antidepressants may develop severe prolonged hypertension. Phenothiazines may reduce or reverse the pressor effect of the epinephrine.

Diphenhydramine hydrochloride (Benadryl®) may be administered to those patients who are allergic to both the ester-type and the amide-type local anesthetics. It may also be given to those persons who have had a documented allergic reaction but the anesthetic agent is unknown. A solution of 50 mg of diphenhydramine hydrochloride (1 ml) should be diluted in 4 ml of normal saline solution for injection. This solution can then be used for local infiltration of wounds and has a duration equivalent to 1% lidocaine plain. It is not recommended for peripheral nerve block anesthesia.

TAC, an acronym for tetracaine, adrenalin, and cocaine was another type of commonly used topical anesthetic used throughout the U.S. through the 1990's. Many cases of adverse reactions, including one well-reported infant death, related to its cocaine component, led to the search for a safer topical anesthetic preparation. As a result, TAC has fallen out of favor with most in the medical community. Caution should always be exercised when using TAC near or around any mucosal membrane or denuded skin.

Topical anesthetic agents such as **LET,** an acronym for lidocaine, epinephrine and tetracaine, can often be as effective as infiltration anesthesia. This anesthetic is well received by pediatric patients because local infiltration is usually not required. As with anesthetics containing epinephrine, care must be exercised when using LET on areas with limited collateral blood supply (i.e., the digits, the tip of the nose, the penis) or where rapid systemic absorption of the drugs is possible (i.e., mucosal membranes). The LET solution or gel is applied to a cotton ball (not gauze) and applied firmly to the wound and the surrounding skin, usually by an adult whose hand is gloved. Anesthesia is achieved in about 20 minutes as evidenced by a blanching of the surrounding skin. If blanching fails or is not complete, local infiltration of the wound edges is necessary before any procedure can proceed.

Many clinical studies have examined the efficacy of **buffering local anesthetics** with sodium bicarbonate solution (1 mEq/ml) to reduce the pain of injection. These studies have shown that the addition of 1 ml of sodium bicarbonate solution to 9 ml of lidocaine is effective in reducing the patient's pain perception. The effect is attributable to buffering the acidic anesthetic solution (pH 6.5) to a more neutral 7.35 pH. However, buffering solutions does reduce the stability of the anesthetic and thereby reduces the shelf life to about 72 hours. Local anesthetic agents containing epinephrine should not be buffered because precipitation of the epinephrine out of the solution will result.

There are some other points to consider when using local anesthetics. Never inject any anesthetic circumferentially around a digit or appendage with a terminal blood supply. In so doing, the neurovascular bundles may be compressed and ischemic changes to the distal tissues may result.

The accidental injection of epinephrine-containing local anesthetics into the digits or end-artery areas has become a relatively common occurrence. Acceptable treatment options have included observation only, the application of warm compresses and wraps, local infiltration of bupivacaine (for its vasodilatory effects), terbutaline infiltration, and transdermal nitroglycerin paste. In more severe instances, the ischemic changes may be reversed by infiltrating **phentolamine mesylate** $(0.5 - 2$ mg of phentolamine diluted in 2 ml of plain lidocaine). The injection can be given either at the puncture site or a digital block may be performed. Even though phentolamine has been used successfully to reverse the α-adrenergic effects of epinephrine, a limited number of clinical reports have been written on the subject. Furthermore, there remains no clear clinical guidelines for its use in this situation.

Finally, care should always be exercised so as not to distort the wound margins when locally infiltrating a wound. For example, this is particularly important in lip lacerations involving the vermilion cutaneous border. Direct infiltration of the lip will distort the margins and make accurate repair difficult. The preferred alternative of anesthetizing this area would be to use an infraorbital or mental nerve block, whichever is most appropriate for the laceration location.

LOCAL ANESTHETIC ADMINISTRATION

Infiltration anesthesia is accomplished by injecting the solution intradermally, subcutaneously, or submucosally across the path of the nerves supplying the injured area.

As a rule, the smallest volume and the lowest concentration of anesthetic solution required to produce the desired effect should be utilized. Of course, this will depend on the anticipated length of the procedure, the degree of anesthesia desired, and the individual patient's response to the anesthetic.

A suitable syringe and needle combination should be used to reduce the discomfort to the patient during injection. For example, if a 10 ml syringe and a 27 gauge needle are used, discomfort to the patient is increased due to the greater hydraulic pressure exerted by this syringe/needle combination. However, a 3 ml syringe / 27 gauge needle combination or a 10 ml syringe / 25 needle combination will make infiltration easier for the provider and less painful for the patient. One can better appreciate the amount of pressure needed for infiltration when following the suggestions above.

Local infiltration techniques vary from infiltration through the wound margins to infiltration through the intact skin surrounding the wound site. Either method is acceptable and effective but infiltrating through the wound margins into the subcutaneous tissue is recommended (Fig. 6.1). However, if the wound is grossly contaminated or infected, a field block or infiltration

Principles of Primary Wound Management

through healthy intact skin may be preferable.

Infiltration through the wound margins is more comfortable for the patient for two reasons. First, visualizing and entering at the level of the subdermal plexus with a fine needle is less painful than puncturing and injecting through intact skin. Second, less injection pressure is required because the subcutaneous tissues are not as dense as the connective tissue of the intact dermis and will accept the anesthetic solution with less effort or pain.

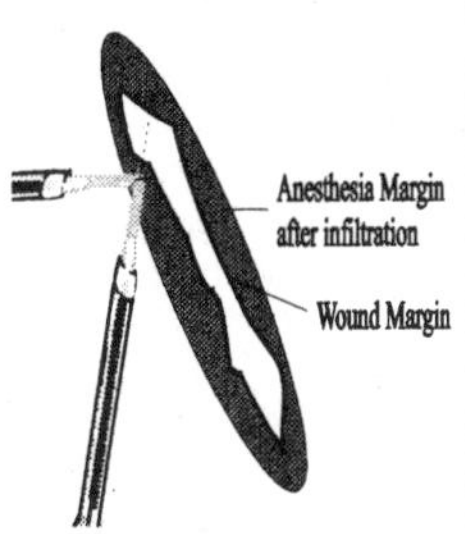

After the needle is inserted into the

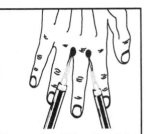

Figure 6.1 Infiltration of local anesthetic through and around wound margin.

wound, aspiration of the syringe plunger should always be performed prior to injection; this will reduce the risk of intravascular injection. Likewise, the plunger should be aspirated before injection anytime the needle is redirected or repositioned. Failure to aspirate blood into the syringe does not guarantee that the needle is not in a vessel. If blood is aspirated, the syringe should be removed from the wound and discarded. A new syringe with local anesthetic is then used to anesthetize the wound.

If an injection must be made through intact skin, one should always wipe the skin with isopropyl alcohol or povidone-iodine solution (unless sensitive or allergic). Swabbing too close to the wound before infiltration may cause significant pain to the patient. Following the skin prep, the needle is quickly inserted into the intact skin and a small wheal of anesthesia is deposited. This technique will allow subsequent painless needle insertions, if necessary, should the patient cause the needle to be withdrawn suddenly during infiltration or for those times when more anesthesia is required.

PERIPHERAL NERVE BLOCK TECHNIQUES

Digital nerve block anesthesia is preferred to direct infiltration of the digits for several reasons. First, the injections are relatively less painful when performed correctly. For example, the tissue at the fingertip lacks the capacity to distend easily to the volume of anesthetic and has sensory nerve endings more closely spaced than the webspace; making the injection more painful in the fingertip. Second, less volume is required to achieve a digital block; 3 ml will block the entire digit. Finally, there is less risk of causing compression of the neurovascular bundle by injecting

Figure 6.2 Webspace digital nerve block of the finger (see first method in text).

through the webspace versus injecting on the digit proper.

Anesthesia by digital block is accomplished by directly injecting an anesthetic **without epinephrine** around or in the vicinity of the proper digital nerves of each digit (fingers or toes). This is done at the level of the metacarpophalangeal joints (MCPJ) or the metatarsophalangeal joints (MTPJ). One should be familiar with the anatomy of the digits with regard to nerve and blood vessel distribution. Although it is not always possible, there should be no deliberate effort to elicit paresthesias or nerve penetration when performing any nerve block.

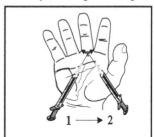

As mentioned earlier, place the patient in a recumbent or supine position before performing any physical manipulation of a wound, including the administration of local anesthesia, wound preparation, and suturing.

Figure 6.3 Digital nerve block of the finger (palmar approach).

There are two commonly-used methods for carrying out digital nerve blocks. The *first method* involves an injection into the webspace on either side of the injured digit (Fig. 6.2). This is the preferred method for a MCP (finger) nerve block and a MTP (toe) nerve block. Before any injection through intact skin, cleanse the skin with either an alcohol swab or povidone-iodine. The needle should be angled slightly volar and toward the metacarpal head of the affected finger. To block the entire digit, injection of 1.5 ml of 2% lidocaine or mepivacaine or 0.25 % (or 0.5%) bupivacaine are required for each side of the digit. Remember NO EPINEPHRINE! Do use a 27 gauge needle and a 3 ml syringe and advise the patient that he may experience numbness of one-half of the adjacent digit(s).

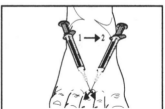

Figure 6.4 Digital nerve block of the toe (see text).

The *second method* of performing a digital nerve block (Fig. 6.3) requires only one injection of the epinephrine-free anesthetic. The same agents as described above may be used. The block is accomplished by injecting 1.5 ml - 2 ml on either side of the metacarpal head from a palmar approach. The first injection is made midway over the volar MCP crease and the needle is directed from one side to the other. Care should be taken to avoid injection into the tendon sheath or the flexor tendon itself. This method can be more painful than the webspace digital block but requires only one needle puncture. Therefore it's use is not recommended for persons with thickly callused palms (i.e., heavy laborers) or for MTP (toe) blocks because of the extreme sensitivity of the plantar skin and the relative non-distensibility of the plantar fascia.

For **toe nerve blocks**, the needle should be inserted dorsally on one side of the extensor tendon at the MTP joint (Fig. 6.4) and then the other. The needle, is advanced in a plantar fashion and the anesthetic deposited adjacent to the digital nerves. The injection of the anesthetic, preceded by aspiration of the syringe plunger, should take place slowly.

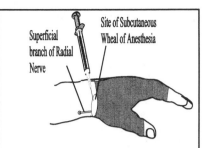

Figure 6.5 Location and innervation of superficial branch of the radial nerve.

Since the thumb is innervated by branches of both the radial and the median nerves, each of those nerves must be blocked individually in order to accomplish a complete **THUMB BLOCK**. The *superficial branch of the radial nerve* (Fig 6.5) is blocked by drawing 3 ml of 2% lidocaine or bupivacaine without epinephrine into a 3 ml syringe. If available use a 27 gauge 1¼" needle and subcutaneously inject over the

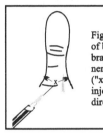

Figure 6.6. Location of block for recurrent branch of the median nerve of the thumb ("x" denotes point of injection; arrows show direction of injection).

distal radius at the level of the distal wrist crease. The subcutaneous wheal of anesthetic should be extended over the dorsum of the wrist toward the extensor carpi radialis longus and brevis tendons. Extreme care should be exercised to prevent an intravascular bolus injection of the anesthetic into the radial artery.

The volar aspect of the thumb and distal phalanx are innervated by the *recurrent branch of the median nerve*. Using 2 ml - 3 ml of 2% lidocaine or bupivacaine without epinephrine and a 27 gauge ½" needle, the anesthetic is placed on either side of the thumb at the level of the MCP crease as shown in Figure 6.6. Remember that the digital nerves of the thumb lie more volar and closer together than those in the fingers.

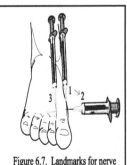

Figure 6.7. Landmarks for nerve block of the great toe (see text).

To perform a **GREAT TOE BLOCK**, one must inject 3 ml - 5 ml of 2% lidocaine or bupivacaine using a 27 gauge 1¼" needle. The first skin puncture is made dorso-medially at the MTP joint of the great toe. The needle is inserted so that the needle is in a dorso-plantar direction almost to the plantar surface (Fig. 6.7). The anesthetic is slowly injected into the skin until a small wheal is palpated on the plantar surface. Without completely withdrawing the needle from the skin, the needle can then be redirected over the dorsum of the great toe toward the lateral border. A small amount of the total anesthesia is injected over the dorsum of the toe. The second needle puncture site is made on the lateral border of the great toe at the MTP joint

in a dorso-plantar direction. The anesthetic is infiltrated in the same fashion as the first injection. As stated earlier, one should avoid injecting circumferentially around a digit (i.e., "ring block") due to the increased risk of vascular compression and potential ischemia to the digit. If an injection is needed on the plantar surface of the great toe, it should be made at a different level.

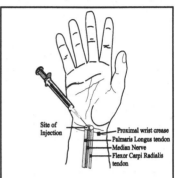

Figure 6.8 Location of landmarks for a median nerve block at the wrist (see text).

WRIST-LEVEL NERVE BLOCKS

Wrist-level nerve blocks enable one to cleanse, inspect, and repair larger lacerations or other injuries to the hand without injecting large volumes of anesthetic solutions.

The procedure for anesthetizing the superficial branch of the radial nerve is discussed in the previous page (see **THUMB BLOCK**).

At the level of the proximal wrist crease, the *median nerve* passes between the tendons of the palmaris longus and the flexor carpi radialis (Fig 6.8). To effectively block the median nerve at this level, one first palpates the palmaris longus and flexor carpi radialis tendons and makes an injection just radial to the palmaris longus tendon.

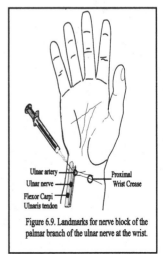

Figure 6.9. Landmarks for nerve block of the palmar branch of the ulnar nerve at the wrist.

The needle is inserted at a 90° angle to the skin at the proximal wrist crease. It is advisable to inject a small subcutaneous wheal of anesthesia immediately after puncturing the skin. This will make any subsequent injections in this area painless.

To complete this block, the needle is inserted through the flexor retinaculum and the anesthetic deposited. A subtle "pop" may be appreciated as the needle passes through the retinaculum. Touching the nerve with the tip of the needle will elicit a paresthesia; causing the patient to pull the hand away or remark that a "tingling or shocking sensation" was felt in the fingers. It is preferable to warn the patient in advance that such a feeling may be experienced. Eliciting a paresthesia should not be the objective but it is sometimes unavoidable. If a paresthesia is elicited, deposit 3 ml of anesthetic around the nerve (not in the nerve) after slightly withdrawing the needle. If no paresthesia is elicited, inject 5 ml below the retinaculum.

It should be noted here that about 15% of the population does not have a palmaris longus tendon. If no palmaris longus tendon is palpated, 3 - 5 ml of 2% lidocaine or bupivacaine without epinephrine should be injected about 1 cm ulnar to the flexor carpi radialis tendon. Wait 20 - 30 minutes for the full effect of this block.

The *ulnar nerve* lies just radial to the flexor carpi ulnaris tendon at the level of the ulnar styloid (Fig 6.9). The palmar branch of the ulnar nerve, which supplies sensation to the hypothenar eminence and the palmar surfaces of the little finger and one-half of the ring finger, lies superficial to the flexor retinaculum. It is blocked by injecting 3 ml of 2% lidocaine or bupivacaine without epinephrine adjacent to the flexor carpi ulnaris tendon. Care should be taken to avoid an intravascular injection into the ulnar artery. The dorsal branch of the ulnar nerve supplies sensation to the dorso-ulnar surface of the hand. The dorsal cutaneous branch of the ulnar nerve is blocked by depositing 3 ml - 5 ml of the same anesthetic subcutaneously around the ulnar styloid from the flexor carpi ulnaris to the dorsum of the hand. The dorsal cutaneous ulnar nerve block is comparable to the superficial radial nerve block in terms of depth and path of injection.

FACIAL NERVE BLOCKS

The most commonly used facial nerve blocks are: 1) the supraorbital and supratrochlear nerve blocks, 2) the infraorbital nerve block, 3) the mental nerve

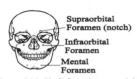

Figure 6.10 Skull foramina essential for facial nerve block landmarks.

block, and 4) the auricular nerve blocks. They provide excellent anesthesia for the cleansing, removal of embedded foreign bodies, and the repair of extensive facial lacerations while keeping the volume of anesthetic to a minimum. When using anesthetics containing epinephrine, one should realize that the addition of a vasoconstrictor only prolongs the duration of the anesthesia and does not provide practical hemostasis when injected anywhere other than the wound margin.

The *supraorbital and supratrochlear nerves* exit through the supraorbital notch on the superior orbital ridge approximately 2.5 cm lateral to the midline of the face. The supratrochlear nerve lies just medial to the supraorbital nerve. Together they supply sensation to the forehead and frontal scalp, from the ipsilateral eyebrow to the coronal suture (Fig. 6.11). To locate these nerves, palpate the supraorbital notch just medial to the midpoint of the eyebrow and use one of the following two methods to achieve successful anesthesia. Bilateral supraorbital and supratrochlear nerve blocks are required to anesthetize the entire forehead and frontal scalp.

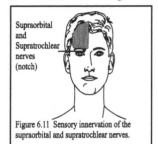

Figure 6.11 Sensory innervation of the supraorbital and supratrochlear nerves.

The *first method* of blocking the supraorbital and supratrochlear nerves requires an injection of 3 ml of 2% lidocaine with epinephrine. After the skin is prepped, the injection is made at the supraorbital notch (while it is palpated) and redirection of the needle 0.5 to 1.0 cm medial to the notch to anesthetize both nerves. Aspiration of the syringe plunger is necessary to reduce the risk of an intravascular

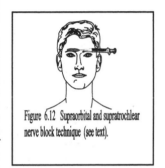

Figure 6.12 Supraorbital and supratrochlear nerve block technique (see text).

injection. Furthermore, care should be exercised to keep the needle parallel to the skin and pointed away from the globe; thus avoiding potential globe penetration should the patient suddenly lift his head.

The *second method* (Fig. 6.12) requires the subcutaneous injection horizontally above the desired eyebrow toward the midline of the face (field block). After the skin is prepped, one can inject a total of 3 ml of lidocaine with epinephrine. The advantage of this method is that virtually all of the branches of the supraorbital and supratrochlear nerves can be blocked without palpating the supraorbital notch or risking globe penetration because the injection is above the bony orbital rim.

The *infraorbital nerve* exits the infraorbital foramen just inferior to the orbital rim. It supplies sensation to the infraorbital region of the cheek, lateral margin of the nasal ala, the ipsilateral upper lip, gingiva, and buccal mucosa (Fig. 6.13). The nerve may be blocked by either an intraoral injection or an

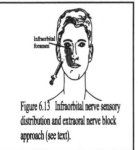

Figure 6.13 Infraorbital nerve sensory distribution and extraoral nerve block approach (see text).

extraoral route. Many believe that the intraoral route is both easy to perform and more comfortable for the patient because skin penetration is not necessary.

The *extraoral approach* to the infraorbital nerve block is attained through the intact skin of the cheek (Fig. 6.13). Following skin preparation, the anesthetic is injected similarly in a small "V"-pattern inferior to the palpated infraorbital foramen. Since the injection is made through intact skin on the face, the patient will experience some discomfort.

The *intraoral approach* to the infraorbital nerve block involves the injection of 2 ml to 2 ½ ml of lidocaine with epinephrine through a 27 gauge needle (preferably 1¼" long). First, palpate the infraorbital foramen on the side to be blocked and mark that point with the index finger. With the patient's mouth open, locate the upper canine tooth, lift the upper lip and inject through the buccogingival fold just medial to the canine tooth. Advance the needle until the tip of the needle is felt beneath the index finger. Aspirate and slowly inject the solution in a small "V"-pattern beneath the finger (about 0.5 cm inferior to the foreman). Gently jiggling the lip during injection can distract the patient from the pain of injection. There is no need to advance the needle to the bone or directly into the foramen since the desired effect is accomplished by placing the anesthetic across the path of the nerve.

The *mental nerve* exits the mental foramen below the second premolar on the mandible and innervates the ipsilateral lower lip, gingiva, buccal mucosa, and skin above the mental protuberance (Fig. 6.14). It does not effectively anesthetize the skin of the submental region.

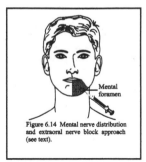

Figure 6.14 Mental nerve distribution and extraoral nerve block approach (see text).

An *extraoral approach* (Fig. 6.14) to the mental nerve block may be used with the same degree of efficacy as the intraoral route but will result in slight increase in patient discomfort secondary to injection through intact skin.

The *intraoral* route of anesthetizing the mental nerve involves injecting 2 - 2½ ml of lidocaine with epinephrine at the base of the second premolar toward the palpated mental foramen will result in excellent and rapid anesthesia (Fig. 6.15). Bilateral mental nerve blocks, sometimes referred to as "puppet" blocks, anesthetize the entire lower lip, mucosa, and skin.

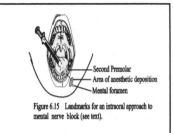

Figure 6.15 Landmarks for an intraoral approach to mental nerve block (see text).

Nerve blockade of one or all of the nerves providing sensation to the *ear* is recommended when infiltration of the wound is difficult or impractical. It is sometimes undesirable to infiltrate due to the close adherence of the skin to the cartilage and subsequent tissue distortion. Nerve block anesthesia is useful for extensive lacerations to the ear but may not be necessary for small wounds.

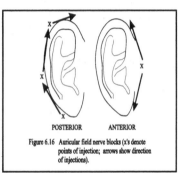

Figure 6.16 Auricular field nerve blocks (x's denote points of injection; arrows show direction of injections).

The *posterior surface of the ear* and much of the external ear canal is innervated by the greater auricular nerve and the lesser occipital nerve. These nerves may be blocked by injecting 3 - 5 ml of 2% lidocaine with epinephrine in a semi-circular fashion behind and at the base of the ear (Fig. 6.16). This injection is best accomplished using a 27 gauge 1¼" needle and injecting subcutaneously where the skin of the posterior surface of the ear meets the skin of the mastoid process.

The auriculotemporal nerve innervates the *anterior and superior surfaces of the ear.* This nerve may be blocked by administering 2 - 3 ml of lidocaine with epinephrine subcutaneously from the lobe to the superior pole of the ear anteriorly (Fig. 6.16). In the event that a small area remains unanesthetized, local infiltration of the area can be carried out. A 1 ml tuberculin (TB) syringe is very useful for the latter injection.

ANKLE-LEVEL NERVE BLOCKS

Although ankle-level nerve blocks are not necessary for most small or simple wound repair, they are very useful in providing anesthesia to large or sensitive areas the foot. Direct infiltration of anesthetics into the plantar surface of the foot is very painful due, in part, to the close adherence of the skin to the dense underlying plantar fascia. Employing nerve blocks at the ankle eliminates the need for large

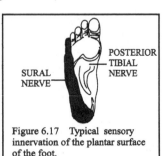

Figure 6.17 Typical sensory innervation of the plantar surface of the foot.

quantities of anesthetic solutions to repair extensive injuries. The use of vasoconstrictors is not recommended for these ankle blocks. Only the most useful ankle-level nerve blocks will be described below: the posterior tibial and the sural nerve blocks. Patients should be advised not to operate a motor vehicle or ambulate without assistance until after the nerve blocks have worn off.

The *posterior tibial nerve*, a branch of the sciatic nerve, supplies sensation to about one-half of the plantar surface of the foot (Fig. 6.17). The nerve lies between the posterior tibial artery and the Achilles tendon posterior to the medial malleolus. To block the posterior tibial nerve, place the patient in a comfortable and prone position. After the skin has been prepped, palpate the posterior tibial artery. The site of injection is the upper border of the medial malleolus between the artery and the Achilles tendon (Fig. 16.18). Approximately 5 - 10 ml of 2% lidocaine or bupivacaine **without** epinephrine should be injected just posterior and lateral to the artery after a small wheal of anesthesia is placed in the skin at the entry site. As always, care should be taken to prevent an intravascular injection by aspirating the plunger of the syringe. Onset of anesthesia and full effect occurs within 15 minutes.

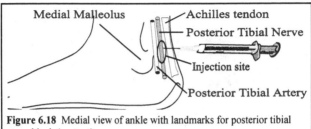

Figure 6.18 Medial view of ankle with landmarks for posterior tibial nerve block (see text).

The *sural nerve*, arising from the common peroneal nerve and a branch of the tibial nerve, supplies sensation to the lateral one-third of the plantar and lateral surfaces of the foot and little toe, as well as the heel (Fig. 6.17). This superficial nerve is blocked by injecting 5 ml of 2% lidocaine or bupivacaine without epinephrine from the superior border of the lateral malleolus to the Achilles tendon (Fig. 16.19).

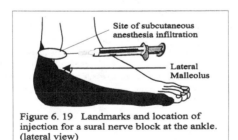

Figure 6. 19 Landmarks and location of injection for a sural nerve block at the ankle. (lateral view)

WOUND PREPARATION TECHNIQUES

After the skin around the wound has been completely anesthetized, the wound and skin adjacent to the wound should be cleansed. Although there are scores of commercial wound preparation trays available, one needs only the following components to cleanse most wounds:

- One Mayo stand or table
- One sterile cloth or polylined paper drape
- One sterile basin (500 - 1000 ml capacity)
- One sterile 30 ml leur lock syringe and a ZeroWet Splashshield **OR**, One sterile 60 ml leur lock syringe and a ZeroWet Splashshield
- One sterile povidone/iodine-soaked sponged (i.e., EZ scrub surgical hand scrub brush with nail cleaner). Do not throw the nail cleaner away; it can be used to retract the wound margin while irrigating.
- About 20 sterile 4x4s
- 500 ml to 1 liter of sterile saline irrigation solution

In the past, many institutions advocated soaking an injured wound (i.e., hand or foot) in a basin of povidone-iodine, hydrogen peroxide, or some other antiseptic solution. Fortunately, this practice in most instances has been discontinued. Numerous laboratory and clinical studies have proven that soaking alone in any solution, other than normal saline or ringers lactate, inhibits normal healing processes and may increase the risk of infection. This occurs partly because the wounds were not irrigated; leaving debris and the cleansing solution in the wound prior to closure. Mere soaking, even in normal saline, does not prevent infection. These studies concluded that when wounds were cleansed with a solution that was not cytotoxic and then irrigated with isotonic saline under pressure, the wounds healed more normally and with fewer complications.

There has been some controversy over the years about which wound cleansing solution is the most beneficial or least cytotoxic. Many have said that solutions that would not be placed in the eye should not be placed in an open wound. It is evident that most investigators and clinicians believe that solutions such as isopropyl alcohol, hydrogen peroxide, chlorhexidine, and hexachlorophene are injurious to healthy tissues. Likewise, deeply pigmented or concentrated solutions make viable tissue identification difficult by staining tissues. In addition, most clinicians have come to realize that no wound prep solution will sterilize a wound. Instead, proper solutions (i.e., polaxamer 188, dilute povidone-iodine) may be used to clean the skin of dirt but this must always be followed by normal saline irrigation under pressure.

As always, the patient should be lying comfortably on a stretcher or bed. To prepare the wound for repair, it is recommended that some sort of absorbent polylined pad (i.e., chux underpad) be placed under the injured area to protect the patient from irrigation and body fluids. One should keep in mind that these pads are not sterile and therefore should not be touched once the provider is sterilely gloved. The use of arm boards is helpful for upper extremity wound procedures.

SKIN PREPARATION

The povidone-iodine soaked sponge previously described should be moistened with sterile saline from the basin. However, the sponge should not be placed into the basin as it will contaminate the normal saline solution to be used for subsequent wound irrigation. The sponge may be moistened by 1) drawing 10 - 15 ml of saline from the basin with a syringe and placing the saline on the sponge or 2) take a saline-soaked 4x4 and squeeze the saline onto the sponge. These simple methods will insure that the wound irrigation solution is saline only and not a mixed solution (povidone-iodine and saline).

Next, take the sponge and gently clean the skin around the wound and up to the wound edges. This gentle but thorough scrub should continue for 2 - 4 minutes, or longer if the skin is heavily contaminated with dirt or grease. A large enough area around the wound should be cleaned to prevent subsequent accidental contamination. For example, clean the whole hand to the wrist even if the patient has only two fingers lacerated. This gives the provider a larger clean field. Scrubbing with the povidone-iodine solution and the sponge is not meant to kill bacteria. Rather, the scrub acts to loosen debris, dirt and bacteria on the skin so it can be irrigated away.

Grease may be removed from the surrounding skin by utilizing an antibacterial ointment (i.e., neosporin, polysporin, bacitracin). These ointments which have an affinity for greases, are applied to the skin and then gently rubbed with a 4x4 gauze or a microporous sponge. Embedded gravel and road dirt may be removed with a sterile, soft-bristled tooth brush. Rough or overly aggressive scrubbing can convert a superficial abrasion into a deep wound with significant tissue destruction. Remember not to replace the used sponge or other contaminated wound prep items onto the wound prep tray.

Once the mechanical portion of the prep (the scrub) is complete, the wound must be irrigated with sterile normal saline. Studies have proven that as few as 10^5 organisms per gram of tissue are capable of causing infection. In addition, that number decreases to as few as 10^2 organisms per gram of tissue when foreign bodies or devitalized tissue remain in the wound. Therefore, the isotonic irrigation solution is used around the wound and then into the wound to remove all soap, blood clots and foreign debris. Adequate splash shielding or protection measures should be utilized. There are several commercially prepared splash device on the market (i.e., Zerowet Splashield®). Several commercial wound irrigation systems allow for irrigation with large volumes of saline directly from a bag of intravenous normal saline solution using a large capacity, spring-loaded syringe (i.e., Irrijet®).

The catheter should never be placed directly into the wound; instead, they should be held about 6 cm from the skin. Advise the patient that the catheter will not touch the skin or cause pain. Saline should be sprayed with adequate pressure (at least 7 - 9 psi) to "blast" the loosened debris from the wound and surrounding skin. The following **minimum** wound irrigation guidelines are recommended:

- If the wound is tidy and clean, 50 ml / cm length and depth
- If the wound is untidy or dirty, 100 ml / cm length and depth

The above recommendations are minimum volumes and frequently more than the minimum is required. This means that if presented with a 5 cm contaminated leg wound a minimum of 500 ml (100 ml / cm x 5 cm = 500 ml) of normal saline should be used to irrigate the wound. Of course, this amount may have to be increased due to an extraordinary amount of contamination, the age of the wound, or a very deep wound.

Upon completion of the scrub and irrigation, the wound is covered with sterile 4x4s. Contamination of the newly cleansed wound and surrounding skin must be avoided. At this point, the provider's gloves must be changed before wound repair proceeds. The wound may now be repaired provided it does not need debridement or excision (see Section 9).

HAIR PREPARATION

The treatment of scalp and facial hair preparation is an important matter to discuss. Hair can be thoroughly cleaned using the same methods described previously for the skin. Hair *does not* need to be shaved prior to repair. The presence of hair does not presume increased infection potential, particularly if properly cleaned. Eyebrow hair should **NEVER** be shaved; doing so will distort the wound edges and make proper alignment of the eyebrow borders difficult, if not impossible. In addition, sometimes shaved eyebrow hair does not grow back or may grow irregularly. Several clinical and laboratory studies have demonstrated that shaving hair well in advance of wound repair actually increases the risk of infection. This occurs because small nicks in the skin from the prep razors or clippers create sites for bacterial colonization. Hair that was shaved just prior to surgery or wound repair was less likely to become infected.

From an aesthetic viewpoint, the practice of shaving scalp or facial hair around a wound site is not appealing. Sutures or staples will have been removed and the wound healed long before the hair that was shaved grows back. Therefore, in most cases, shaving hair is only for the convenience of the provider and not the patient.

However, this is not to say that there aren't indications or occasions that warrant shaving hair. One may have a patient with an extensive scalp laceration or numerous wounds that cannot be adequately visualized unless hair is removed. Excessive hair removal may be unsightly and may distort anatomical landmarks or borders; making repair difficult. If hair must be removed, only shave approximately 1 cm around the wound.

Many healthcare providers have argued that hair must be shaved to keep it from becoming entangled in the sutures or the wound itself. This so-called "problem" can be solved by taking a few extra seconds at the end of the procedure to remove the hair from the knotted sutures or from within the wound margins. One only needs to pull the hair from these sites using fingers, forceps, or the closed points of the iris scissors and the "problem" is solved.

There are two commonly used alternatives to shaving hair. First, consider using a lubricating jelly or antibiotic ointment to the prepped hair adjacent to the wound site. The jelly or ointment can be placed on the hair to keep it flat and out of the provider's field during repair. Furthermore, these substances may be washed out of the hair by the patient beginning the next day. Bacitracin or similar ointments are very greasy and when applied heavily may take a few days to wash out of the hair. For most patients, however, washing ointment out of hair is preferable to having a bald spot.

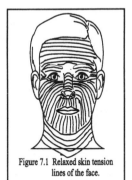

Figure 7.1 Relaxed skin tension lines of the face.

The second alternative to shaving is trimming the hair immediately around the wound to approximately 0.5 cm in length. This will eliminate nicks in the skin and bald spots but will leave a short stubble and make suture handling easier.

WOUND DEBRIDEMENT AND EXCISION

Debridement is the removal of dead or contaminated tissue to provide better approximation, a better cosmetic result, and lessen the likelihood of infection. This should be done without damaging underlying vital structures. Some areas of the body, such as the face, lend themselves to extensive debridement more readily than do areas where there is little redundant tissue (i.e., the hand, fingers, toes). In most instances, debridement should be limited to no more than a couple of millimeters from the wound edge. If too much tissue is debrided or excised, or the procedure

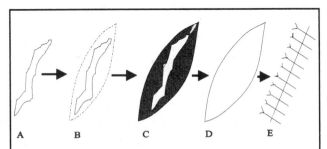

Figure 7.2 Wound excision technique. A, untidy wound; B, wound with light "marking" incision around margins; C, shaded area represents tissue to be removed; D, "new" wound with fresh margins; E, sutured wound (see text).

is performed incorrectly, the newly created defect may be worse than the original injury.

Before making any incision, the provider must be aware of the skin tension patterns and the underlying anatomy. The skin tension lines of the face are illustrated in Figure 7.1. To make it easier to remember, these lines are perpendicular to the fibers of the underlying muscles.

The procedures for debriding devitalized tissue are relatively simple, but must be carefully planned before starting. The selection of one of the methods below depends upon how much tissue needs to be removed.

Debridement involves the use of sharp iris scissors and is intended to remove a small amount of tissue from the wound margins. One should trim the wound margins a millimeter or two to get rid of the thin epidermal or irregular edges.

Excision is a surgical method used to revise large, untidy wounds or remove skin lesions. Excision requires sharp tissue dissection with a #15 scalpel blade followed by tissue removal using iris scissors and Adson forceps with teeth. The length of the ellipsoid incision should be at least 3 times the wound width. Incisions less than 3 times the width will result in a dog-ear deformity.

With firm tension applied by one's fingers along the wound axis, a light "marking" incision is made into the dermis (Fig 7.2B) usually following the shape of the wound and, when possible, the skin tension lines. The skin should bleed only slightly after the "marking" incision is made. The purpose of the "marking" incision is to allow the provider a path to follow when removing the tissue. Once the "marking" incision is made, the devitalized tissue inside the marking incision can be grasped with the forceps (Fig. 7.2C). Iris scissors, or a scalpel, are now used to trim away the devitalized tissue down to the subcutaneous fat. The resulting wound margins (Fig. 7.2D) should be made as perpendicular to the skin surface as possible to facilitate easier wound margin apposition (Fig 7.3). This procedure is repeated on the other wound margin. Any necrotic or contaminated fat

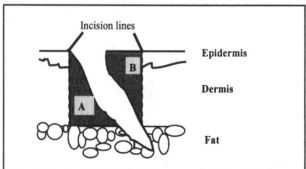

Figure 7.3   Repair of a full-thickness wound with beveled edges. "A" and "B" are debrided after a perpendicular incision is made into the dermis and only to the subcutaneous fat. Undermining may be necessary to achieve a tension-free wound closure.

Principles of Primary Wound Management

should be debrided before closure. As a general rule, viable tissue bleeds readily and nonviable tissue does not. Removing too much of the underlying support for the skin may lead to complications, such as scar depression. After excision is complete, the wound can be repaired (Fig. 7.2E).

Damage to all underlying nerves, blood vessels, muscles, and tendons must be avoided when performing either of the above techniques. Blunt dissection, rather than sharp dissection, around blood vessels and nerves is strongly recommended. Maintaining a near bloodless operating field is a necessity in such situations. This can be accomplished with the use of epinephrine in the anesthetic (except where contraindicated), direct pressure, or a tourniquet. If debridement procedures run the risk of injuring any vital structure, it may be best to forego debridement altogether, repair the wound, and have the patient follow up with a plastic surgeon for later wound revision.

UNDERMINING TISSUE

After the debridement procedures are complete and the wound is found to be under too much tension for easy apposition, undermining may be necessary for proper wound closure. Undermining is simply the careful separation of one tissue layer from another to allow for easier wound margin apposition. The wound should be undermined approximately the width of the wound along both margins and at the corners. It also minimizes tension on the edges during healing. The procedure involves the blunt separation of the dermis from the subcutaneous fat or muscle using iris or Mayo scissors. As always, care should be exercised so as not to damage blood vessels or nerves.

Please note that not all wounds that appear wide require undermining. If the skin can be easily apposed with intradermal sutures, then undermining is not required.

HEMOSTASIS

A near-bloodless operating field should be maintained to assure maximum visualization of the wound and the underlying anatomy during inspection and repair. Hemostasis during preparation is usually impossible to achieve unless a tourniquet is used. During wound preparation the constant disturbance of tissues and removal of small blood clots promotes bleeding. When anesthetics containing epinephrine are used, the maximal vasoconstrictor effect on the local vasculature is seen within 10 minutes.

In areas where epinephrine use is contraindicated, some sort of tourniquet may be useful to maintain hemostasis. In most cases though, tourniquets are not necessary and their use should be limited. If a tourniquet must be used, the pneumatic-type tourniquet is preferred because the pressure can be accurately controlled. An alternative to this device is the standard sphygmomanometer (blood pressure cuff). The patient's arm or leg may be wrapped with padding (i.e., cast underpadding) and then the cuff is inflated about 100 mm Hg above the patient's systolic blood pressure. When the desired pressure is attained, both cuff tubes must be clamped to prevent the cuff from deflating. Tourniquets are not tolerated for long periods of time unless the entire extremity is anesthetized. Most patients may only remain comfortable and cooperative for 10 minutes with this type of device in place.

Digital tourniquets, approximately ½-inch in thickness, may be used for short periods of time. Tight application or prolonged used of narrow tubing or tourniquets may produce ischemic changes or a neurapraxia in the digit. Digital tourniquets when used with a digital nerve block are tolerated well and can be used up to 30 minutes. Rubber bands, string, or narrow tubing should *never* be used as tourniquets because they can damage the neurovascular bundles or may be forgotten and incorporated into the bandage. If arterial hemostasis is not possible using the methods just described, then a surgical consultation would be in order.

WOUND CLOSURE MATERIALS

When the decision has been made to close a wound, one must select the appropriate suture material to achieve the best possible results. This choice depends upon several factors, including whether or not the wound is under tension or aligned against skin tension lines, whether the wound is at high risk of infection, patient comfort and ease of care, and the anatomical location of the wound.

Many healthcare providers rely solely on what material another person uses "all the time" and they often ignore (or forget) to take into consideration the advantages and disadvantages of the various closure materials. For instance, if the provider is not familiar with the types of suture materials and needles available, the incorrect size (diameter) may be selected for a particular wound closure. Suture size, needle size, handling characteristics, and color of the suture material are especially important when a cosmetic result is required.

SUTURE MATERIALS

All suture materials, regardless of their composition, are foreign bodies when placed into any tissue. In light of this fact, suture bulk or mass should be kept to a minimum. The body reacts to and attempts to degrade the suture by phagocytic, enzymatic or hydrolytic activity.

Suture materials are divided into two groups: absorbable and nonabsorbable sutures (Table 8.1). Each suture in these two groups may be characterized by its relative tissue reactivity, handling features, and composition. In addition, the absorbable sutures are also characterized by their absorption, tensile strength retention, and whether they are braided or monofilament materials.

All sutures which are digested by enzymes or hydrolyzed by tissue fluids are considered absorbable or temporary. An absorbable suture is defined by the United States Pharmacopeia (U.S.P.) as a "sterile strand from collagen derived from healthy mammals or a synthetic polymer. It is capable of being absorbed by living mammalian tissue, but may be treated to modify its resistance to absorption. It may be impregnated or coated with a suitable antimicrobial agent. It may be colored by a

Table 8.1 Suture Reactivity (least to most reactive)

Absorbable Sutures

Polydioxanone (PDS II)
Polyglactin 910 (Vicryl)
Polyglycolic acid (PGA)
Poliglecaprone 25 (Monocryl)
Chromic gut
Plain gut
Fast-absorbing plain gut

Nonabsorbable Sutures

Polypropylene (Prolene)
Nylon
Polyester
Silk

color additive approved by the Food and Drug Administration.". The most commonly used absorbable suture materials are fast-absorbing plain gut, plain gut, chromic gut, polyglactin 910 or polyglycolic acid, poliglecaprone 25, and polydioxanone. The first three materials are natural collagen substances. Polyglactin 910, polyglycolic acid, poliglecaprone 25, and polydioxanone are synthetic absorbable materials.

The absorption times for absorbable suture material vary from tissue to tissue. Tensile strength, retention and absorption rates are independent

Table 8.2 Absorption and Retention Profiles for Absorbable Sutures

Absorbable Suture Type	Total Absorption Time (days) [1]	Retention Time of 50% Tensile Strength (days)
Plain Gut: Fast-absorbing Regular	21 - 42 days [2] 70 days [2]	3 - 4 days [2] 7 - 10 days [2]
Chromic Gut	60 - 90 days [2]	21 - 30 days [2]
Polyglactin 910 coated Vicryl Vicryl *RAPIDE*	90 - 120 days 42 days	21 days 5 days
Polydioxanone (PDS II)	180 days	30 days

[1] Times are for implanted suture material.

[2] Absorption and tensile strength times are shortened in the presence of infection.

events. For example, a suture can lose its tensile strength quickly but be absorbed slowly, or vice versa. Table 8.2 summarizes the average total absorption and tensile strength times for common absorbable sutures.

Any material that is resistant to tissue enzymes and cannot be dissolved is considered nonabsorbable or permanent. When used internally, these materials are encapsulated by fibrous tissue instead of being digested. When used percutaneously, they must be removed to prevent unnecessary and

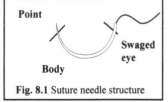

Fig. 8.1 Suture needle structure

unsightly scarring. Examples of nonabsorbable suture materials are: nylon, polypropylene, polyester, silk, and surgical stainless steel.

Sutures have standardized specifications set forth by government regulations. The size of the suture strand refers to the diameter of that strand. A standard nomenclature has been assigned to differentiate between the different sizes of sutures. Zeroes (0's) designate the size of the strand. As the number of zeroes increases, the diameter of the suture strand becomes smaller. For example, a "6-0" (shorthand for 000000) strand is smaller than a "4-0" strand. In addition, the tensile strength decreases as the diameter of the suture decreases. Larger sutures are designated as "1", "2", etc. Table 8.3 reviews the handling characteristics and common indications for the most commonly used suture material.

The proper selection of surgical needles is as important as proper material selection. The three basic sections of the atraumatic needle are: the swaged eye, the body and the point (Fig. 8.1). An atraumatic needle is designed to reduce the amount of tissue trauma as the needle passes through the skin. The diameter of the strand may be available on a variety of needle sizes, designs and radii.

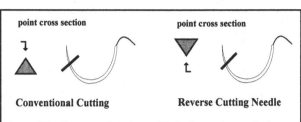

point cross section   **point cross section**

Conventional Cutting   **Reverse Cutting Needle**

Figure 8.2   Suture needle points and body shapes. Arrows depict location of needle cutting surface on cross-section through needle point.

When suturing in the emergency department, office or clinic, either a conventional or reverse cutting needle is used (Fig. 8.2). Some fragile tissues may require taper point needles (similar to an upholstery needle) but their use is primarily limited to the operating room.

TISSUE ADHESIVES

Tissue adhesives received FDA approval in 1998 for human use in the United States. DERMABOND® (2-octyl cyanoacrylate) is a liquid topical skin adhesive that has been marketed as a substititue for sutures and staples in the closure of traumatic wounds. It can also act as a barrier against common bacterial microbes.

DERMABOND® should only be used to hold dry skin (epidermal) edges together. It may be used in conjunction with, but not in the place of, subcuticular sutures. It should not be placed between the wound margins. Likewise, it should not be used on the following: 1) mucosal membranes, 2) heavy hair-bearing areas, 3) actively infected or gangrenous areas, 4) areas exposed to moisture or bodily fluids, and 5) areas of high skin tension (joints) unless they are splinted during healing. Although no formal studies have been done involving the use of DERMABOND® on bite and stab wounds, such wounds should be thoroughly cleansed and allowed to heal secondarily. It should not be used on patients with a known hypersensitivity to cyanoacrylate or formaldehyde.

The manufacturer cites research studies that state DERMABOND® use results in excellent cosmetic results ("similar to those of suturing"), is less likely to require anesthesia, results in less pain, lowers costs, provides faster healing times, eliminates the need for suture removal, and will not produce suture or "track" marks.

Care should be used when using, or contemplating it use around the eyes. Avoid getting DERMABOND® in the eye. Position the patient to allow the adhesive to run away from the eye. Application of an ophthalmic ointment to the eyelashes *prior* to the use of DERMABOND® for eyelid lacerations is suggested to prevent gluing the eyelashes together.

Despite the claims of the manufacturer, the patient's welfare must always come first. It is truthful to say that gluing the skin edges together is much faster and more comfortable than placing sutures or staples in many instances. But getting the patient "in and out" of the office or emergency departement as quickly as possible should not be the primary concern. For all but the most superficial of wounds, careful and accurate wound preparation and closure, following local anesthesia, is necessary. Some practitioners have been quick to use adhesives on crying children instead of considering or performing a layered repair when necessary. Proper wound management skills, including appropriate restraint and / or sedation, may be required to achieve good results. Sutures, when left in the skin too long, will leave suture marks but removing them in a timely fashion can avoid this problem.

Many clinicians have reported and voiced concerns about the physical properties and application characteristics of DERMABOND® over the last few years. The main issues have been the low viscosity and the difficulty of application. The low viscosity of the product has resulted in the adhesive inadvertently running onto adjacent skin areas. A new HIGH VISCOSITY DERMABOND® was created in an attempt to correct the low viscosity issue. This new formulation, six times thicker than the original, is an improvement but it has met with mixed reviews by many clinicians.

The applicator tip (whether the round or chisel types) continues to pose an accurate placement problem during the application. Some clinicians continue to glue their fingers / gloves to the skin while others have difficulty visualizing the wound because their fingers are too close to the wound margins. Many practitioners have devised alternative methods to apply the adhesive. One method involves cracking the ampule and then inserting a fine needle on a tuberculin syringe to draw up the adhesive. Once the adhesive is in the syringe, it can be applied to the skin in a more controlled fashion – drop by drop. Additionally, the development of skin adhesive aids, such as TruLine® wound closure forceps, has helped practitioners visualize the wound better and apply the adhesive without getting fingers in the way.

Aftercare instructions allow the patient to bathe but direct rubbing, scratching or soaking of the repaired area is discouraged. Likewise, the application of ointments or additional bandages over the adhesive is not required. DERMABOND® is expected to break apart and fall off in about 5-10 days after application.

Table 8.3 Handling Characteristics and Uses for Suture Materials

Type of Suture Material	Indications for Suture Use	Comments
ABSORBABLES **Plain Gut: Regular**	Vascular ligation Intraoral laceration repair	Ideal for repair where infection potential is high. Monofilament; bristle-like knot.
Fast-absorbing (FAPG)	**Only for skin repair - NEVER for internal tissues!** Ideal for repair of facial wounds on children.	Rinse FAPG suture strand gently with saline before using; removes some preservative residue.
Chromic Gut	Vascular ligation Muscle repair, Dermal approximation	Same as above
Polyglactin 910/ PGA: **Coated Vicryl ™** **Vicryl *RAPIDE* ™**	Muscle repair and dermal approximation Skin and mucosal repair	Used in tissues with low infection potential and wounds closed without tension. Braided, soft knots. Same as above but can be used for nonfacial skin closure.
Polydioxanone (PDS II ™)	Muscle repair and dermal approximation	Same as above except monofilament. Bristle-like knot.
NONABSORBABLES **Silk**	Intraoral lacerations, eyelid laceration at gray line repair	Braided, very soft knot. Elicits moderate to high tissue reaction due to natural protein composition. Braid "wicks"
Polyester	Same as above	Same as above for handling. Less tissue reaction because synthetic material.
Nylon	Primarily for percutaneous (skin) closure.	Black monofilament. Bristle-like knot. Relatively inert.
Polypropylene (Prolene™)	Primarily for percutaneous (skin) closure. Also used for tendon repair.	Blue monofilament. Bristle-like knot. Ideal for dark-haired or skin areas. Inert.

STAPLES

Stapling is a rapid method of wound repair. Generally, stapling has been reserved for long, linear lacerations of the scalp, extremity and torso. *Staples should not be used for the closure of facial wounds.* The surgical stainless steel staples cause very little tissue reactivity. Although staple placement is rapid and easy, it can result in a less than meticulous closure. Care must be exercised to evert the edges for proper placement and healing. The staples may also interfer with some CT and MRI imaging. Staple removal is simple but it requires a special staple remover. One might consider giving the patient a staple remover if the patient will seek removal at another facility or office.

SECTION 9

BASIC SUTURING PRINCIPLES

Suturing serves four basic purposes: 1) achieves hemostasis, 2) speeds wound healing, 3) decreases risk of wound infection, and 4) generally affords a better cosmetic result. These results are accomplished only when proper suture technique is skillfully and conscientiously employed.

The basic suture tray for general and cosmetic laceration repair should consist of the following instruments: one Webster-type needle holder, one iris scissors, one Adson forceps with 2:1 mouse teeth, one mosquito hemostat, 2 - 4 cloth or paper drapes, and 20 sterile 4x4 gauze sponges.

There are several recognized ways for handling surgical instruments. The "best" method of instrument handling is one that feels comfortable for the   provider and allows complete control and accurate suture placement.

The basic tenets of wound care and suturing are:

1   Be precise - not careless. Take your time.
2   Have good lighting on the wound and the operating field. Be seated and comfortable whenever possible.
3   Repair all layers that have been lacerated, such as the galea, the muscle or fascia, the dermis, and the skin.
4   Evert the wound edges. Avoid wound edge inversion.
5   Approximate the tissue edges without strangulation of the tissue. Do not tie the sutures too tightly.
6   Begin suturing either from one end to the other or use the "halving" technique. Whichever technique is utilized, do not create a dog-ear or leave gaps between the sutures.
7   Always use gentle tissue handling techniques.
8   Minimize the number of suture needle punctures through the skin with each bite.
9   Use only the smallest diameter suture acceptable to achieve the result.
10   Begin each bite with the needle point perpendicular to the skin surface.
11   Follow the arc of the needle. Guide the needle and let it work for you.
12   Make all suture bites equidistant from the wound edge and each adjacent suture.
13   Tie a secure, flat knot. Check knot security. Pull knots off to the side of the wound margin. Make sure the "tails" do not fall into the wound.
14   Keep the number of sutures to a minimum. This varies with the type of tissue and anatomical location being repaired.
15   KNOW YOUR LIMITATIONS AND KNOW WHEN TO DEFER.

Although there are no absolute rules dictating the exact number of sutures necessary for wound closure or what type of suture material must be used, the guidelines found in Table 9.1 will be quite helpful.

Wide scarring can be reduced in most instances by performing a layered closure. This will eliminate dead tissue spaces, prevent hematoma formation, restore function to lacerated tissues (muscle, dermis), and speed

Table 9.1 Recommended Closure Guidelines by Anatomic Location and Tissue Layer

ANATOMICAL WOUND LOCATION	TISSUE LAYER TO BE SUTURED	SUTURE MATERIAL RECOMMENDATION	SUTURE TECHNIQUE
FACE AND NECK	SKIN	6-0 FAPG*, NYLON, POLYPROPYLENE	SIMPLE
	DERMIS	6-0, 5-0 VICRYL, PDS	INVERTED
	MUSCLE	4-0, 5-0 VICRYL, PDS	SIMPLE
	PERICHONDRIUM	6-0 VICRYL	SIMPLE
MOUTH	TONGUE	4-0, 5-0 VICRYL or *RAPIDE*, CHROMIC	SIMPLE; INVERTED
	MUCOSA	SAME AS ABOVE	SIMPLE; INVERTED
SCALP	SKIN	4-0 NYLON, *RAPIDE,* or POLYPROPYLENE	SIMPLE
	DERMIS	4-0 VICRYL, PDS	INVERTED
	MUSCLE, GALEA	3-0, 4-0 VICRYL, PDS	SIMPLE
ARMS AND LEGS (except hands and feet)	SKIN	4-0, 5-0 NYLON, POLYPROPYLENE	SIMPLE; MATTRESS
	DERMIS	4-0, 5-0 VICRYL, PDS	INVERTED
	FASCIA	3-0, 4-0 VICRYL, PDS	SIMPLE
HANDS	SKIN	5-0 NYLON, POLYPROPYLENE	SIMPLE
	NAILBED	6-0 VICRYL	SIMPLE
	DERMIS, FASCIA	5-0 VICRYL; NOTHING IN FINGERS	INVERTED
FEET	SKIN (DORSUM)	4-0, 5-0 NYLON, POLYPROPYLENE	SIMPLE; MATTRESS
	(PLANTAR)	4-0, 5-0 NYLON, POLYPROPYLENE	SIMPLE
	NAILBED	6-0 VICRYL,	SIMPLE
	DERMIS, FASCIA	5-0 VICRYL; NOTHING IN TOES	INVERTED

* FAPG = fast-absorbing plain gut
Simple = simple interrupted loop suture
Inverted = Inverted loop (intradermal) suture

Mattress = horizontal or vertical mattress suture
RAPIDE = *VICRYL RAPIDE*®

wound healing. With the placement of intradermal sutures, wound healing processes proceed with less tension on the skin surface and the collagen-rich dermis. Furthermore, proper suture selection and technique allows the wound margins to remain apposed until collagen synthesis is complete.

Usually, a **general closure** refers to the wound margins (skin and subcutaneous tissues) being approximated with percutaneous sutures and, if necessary, subcutaneous sutures. All percutaneous sutures are positioned close enough together to prevent gaps in the wound margin. The distance between each percutaneous suture varies and is sometimes 3 - 5 mm (i.e., hand, arm) or 5 -10 mm (scalp).

A **cosmetic layered closure**, on the other hand, **requires** subcuticular sutures (i.e., in the dermis, muscle or fascia) and percutaneous sutures placed 2 - 3 mm apart from each other. A cosmetic repair is not limited to facial wound repair. For example, a patient may present to the emergency department with a 4 cm forearm laceration extending through the subcutaneous fat. Such a wound should not be closed in one layer as the margins will most likely "drift" apart over time. The dermis and the skin must be approximated to render a narrower scar. As mentioned earlier, wider scars are often result of failure to close deep wounds in layers or improper suture material selection (i.e., a suture that absorbs too rapidly to provide needed long-term tissue support).

Wound edges must be **everted** in order to allow for faster wound healing and better cosmetic results. Inversion refers to the epidermis falling in between the wound margins during wound repair. While suture or staples are in place, the suture line may appear fine. But after the sutures or staples are removed, the wound margins dehisce. Now the wound is required to heal be secondary intention. Too wide and or too shallow tissue bites or tightly tied sutures lead to wound edge inversion.

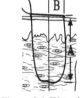

Figure 9.1 Wound eversion technique; A > B = Eversion

There are several ways to achieve wound edge eversion. First, place the needle near one wound margin, enter the skin perpendicular to the surface, and take more tissue at the bottom of the suture path than at the top - go deeper than wide (see Fig. 9.1). The suture needle then enters the opposite wound margin at the same tissue level to avoid a "step-off" of the wound margin as seen from the surface. The entry/exit bites and the depth of the suture bite vary by anatomical location; the placement is different on the scalp versus the eyelid.

Another method to accomplish wound margin eversion is to place either horizontal or vertical mattress sutures in the tissue. These sutures when correctly executed will automatically evert the tissue. They are ideal for any area in which there is excess or redundant tissue (i.e., the elbow, the dorsum of the hand or foot, the webspaces) or areas under stress (i.e., knee). Mattress sutures, however, should **never** be used on the face - *use only simple interrupted sutures for the percutaneous approximation of facial skin.*

All subcutaneous sutures (i.e., intradermal, buried simple interrupted)

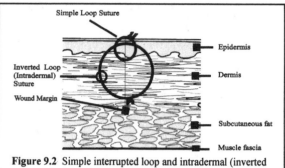

Figure 9.2 Simple interrupted loop and intradermal (inverted loop) suture placement.

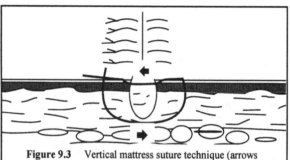

Figure 9.3 Vertical mattress suture technique (arrows indicate direction of suture bite).

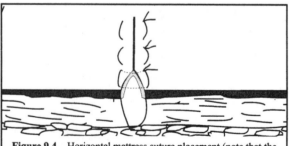

Figure 9.4 Horizontal mattress suture placement (note that the suture bites are placed only through the dermis on both margins).

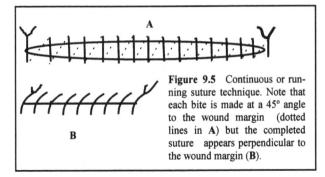

Figure 9.5 Continuous or running suture technique. Note that each bite is made at a 45° angle to the wound margin (dotted lines in **A**) but the completed suture appears perpendicular to the wound margin (**B**).

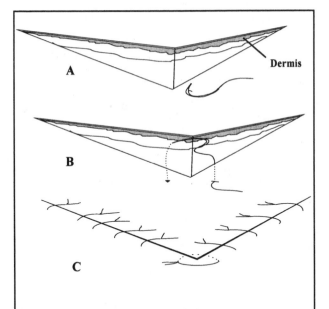

Figure 9.6 Flap or half-buried horizontal mattress suture. **A**, enter skin on non-flap side near apex; **B**, pass the needle through apex of flap into the dermis taking care not to crush the tissue at the apex; **C**, bring suture out of the skin on the non-flap side adjacent to the entry point and tie suture. Note: All passes should be made through the same tissue layer (dermis). This prevents a step-off of the apex margins.

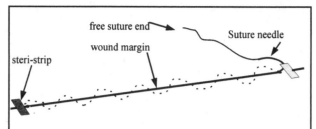

Figure 9.7 Running subcuticular suture placement. Illustrates entry point of needle and suture placement in dermis (dashed lines) over length of wound. Note: secure the free suture ends to the skin with steri-strips.

should not have long suture "tails" left in the wound. The free ends of the sutures should be carefully cut just above the knot. Care should also be taken not to clamp or crimp the monofilament, absorbable suture strands with the needleholders. This weakens the strand and causes premature loss of tensile strength and breakage.

Fatty tissue and skeletal muscle generally do not hold sutures effectively. Sutures placed in the subcutaneous fat will cause necrosis of the fat around each suture. In addition, the suture will remain as a foreign body until it is completely absorbed and will not add to the structural integrity of the healing wound. Instead, sutures should be placed into the collagen-rich muscle fascia and the dermal layers to reapproximate the muscle and subcutaneous fat, respectively.

An exception to the practice of not suturing muscle directly involves the repair of lacerated facial muscles. Facial muscles have very little, if any, visible fascia and therefore they must be repaired carefully by suturing one margin of the muscle to the other. Failure to repair muscle lacerations will result in a poorly functioning muscle, as well as a depressed, unsightly scar.

WOUND DRESSINGS

In general, nonfacial wound dressings consist of three layers:

- The contact layer - single thickness only of xeroform, adaptic, etc.
- The absorbent layer - (i.e., 4x4's, 2x2's)
- The outer layer - (i.e., roll gauze, tube gauze, ace wrap, splint)

Nonfacial wounds should be covered following the recommendations above. There are some points to make about dressing any wound. Be careful not to make the wound dressing too occlusive. Many studies have shown that a slightly moist wound promotes wound healing. However, heavy application of ointment, followed by multiple layers of non-adhering gauze, and finally a bulky wrap will more than likely result in wound maceration. Maceration, or the retention of excessive moisture on and in the skin, can lead to the tracking of bacteria into the wound, wound dehiscence, or wound infection. The use of nonstick pads (i.e., Telfa®) should be avoided. When such pads are left in place too long or if there is excessive moisture (i.e., perspiration), they trap moisture and exudates and cause skin maceration.

In most cases facial wounds do not require bulky dressings. Instead, they only need an antibacterial ointment applied over the wound and possibly a bandaid. If there is the potential for hematoma formation, a compression (pressure) dressing should be used for 1 - 3 days. The bandage should be firmly applied but never tight.

GENERAL FOLLOW-UP CARE GUIDELINES

1   An injured extremity should be kept elevated above heart level for at least 48 hours following injury.

2   If edema is anticipated, cold compresses should be used for 24 - 48 hours (20 - 30 minutes at a time; 4 - 6 times a day).

3   Nonfacial wounds should be dressed with a bulky dressing for the first 24 - 48 hours. Thereafter, they may be washed with soap and water several times a day.

4   If the dressing becomes wet or dirty, it should be removed and the wound should be cleaned with soap and water and redressed.

5   Healing wounds should not be immersed or soaked in water or chemicals. The only possible exception would be to soak an adhering dressing off with half-strength hydrogen peroxide (i.e., after a nail bed repair).

6   Facial wounds should be gently cleansed with mild soap and water 6 or more times a day beginning 24 hours after repair. Alcohol and hydrogen peroxide are usually not necessary. The use of hydrogen peroxide causes a serosanguinous exudate and crust that alarms some patients.

7   Polysporin, bacitracin, or neosporin ointment should be applied to all facial wounds in a thin layer after each cleansing.

8   Healing wounds, particularly facial wounds, need protection from strong sun exposure / sunburn for 8 - 12 months. Sun avoidance or the use of a sunblock with a sun protection factor (SPF) of 15 or higher will usually afford protection and prevent hyperpigmentation of the new scar.

9   All patients should be instructed to observe for the presence of infection: worsening pain, purulent drainage, swelling, fever, chills, red streaking, or the presence of tender / palpable lymph nodes.

10   The patient should be given specific written follow-up instructions for wound checks, suture removal, or specialist referrals.

11   Advise patients that all wounds scar. Some wounds are easily concealed, others are more noticeable because of location, direction and length. When a wound is properly closed (proper materials and technique), the resultant scar should be as narrow. Length cannot be changed; the wound cannot be made shorter with initial suturing.

SUTURE REMOVAL GUIDELINES AND TECHNIQUES

Suture should be removed according to the guidelines found below in Table 9.2. Timely removal will lessen the likelihood of suture abscess formation, cross-hatching or "railroad track" scarring.

Suture removal times vary depending upon the size and depth of the wound, whether there was a multi-layered or single-layered repair, the general health of the patient, the presence of infection or other complications, and patient compliance to the follow-up instructions.

Although suture removal is a very simple procedure, one must make sure that no suture fragments are left behind in the wound. The skin should be lightly cleaned with an alcohol prep pad before removing any sutures.

To remove a simple interrupted (loop) suture, one lifts up on the knot and snips the suture on one side under the knot using a pair of iris scissors or a #11 scalpel blade. The entire suture strand is easily removed from the skin (Fig. 9.7 A). Do not cut both strands under the knot.

Continuous loop (running) sutures are removed by cutting ONE strand under the knot at both ends, similar to the simple interrupted suture removal. After each end is cut, the suture strand may be cut again in thirds if it is long. Care should be exercised to remove all free loops and strands (Fig. 9.7 B). Horizontal mattress sutures may be removed by cutting one strand under the knot or by cutting the suture in half (opposite the knot). The suture is then pulled through the skin (Fig. 9.7 C).

To remove a vertical mattress suture, the strand is cut closest to the skin under the knot and removed (Fig. 9.7 D).

Table 9.2 Suture Removal Guidelines

Wound Location	Removal Times
Facial	3 - 5 days*
Scalp	5 - 8 days
Neck	3 - 5 days*
Chest	7 - 10 days*
Abdomen	7 - 10 days*
Back	10 - 12 days*
Upper Extremity	
Non-joint surface	7 - 10 days*
Joint surface	10 -12 days*
Lower Extremity	
Thigh	7 - 10 days*
Knee	12 - 14 days*
Lower leg	7 - 10 days*
Foot	7 - 10 days*

* followed by tape application on non-hairy areas

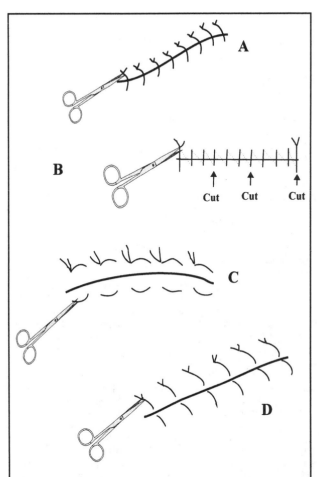

Figures 9.7 A-D. Suture removal techniques. **A,** Simple loop removal; **B,** Continuous loop or running suture removal; **C,** Horizontal mattress suture removal; and **D,** Vertical mattress suture removal (see text).

SPECIFIC WOUND MANAGEMENT PROBLEMS

FACIAL WOUNDS

Most **periorbital lacerations** occur from blunt force trauma (i.e., fists, bottles, broken eyeglasses) and involve the supraorbital ridge and eyelids. The orbicularis oculi muscle, if lacerated, must be repaired with 5-0 polyglactin 910 or polydioxinone. Eyebrow lacerations are sutured in the manner previously discussed (see Table 9.1). Eyebrow wounds do not lend themselves to extensive debridement. However when debridement is indicated, it may be performed on the non-hairy area superior and inferior to the eyebrow borders. Eyebrow hair should not be shaved as it will distort the landmarks needed during repair; thus leaving the patient with an unattractive scar and uneven hair growth.

Superficial or full-thickness lacerations to the eyelid should be closed with 6-0 or 7-0 nylon or polypropylene suture for the skin and/or 5-0 or 6-0 vicryl or polydioxinone for the dermis. Special attention to wound margin eversion is necessary.

Deep punctures or penetrating lacerations to the lids, between the orbital rim and the tarsal plate, must be carefully inspected for injury to the globe and the presence of periorbital fat in the wound. Periorbital fat, or fat surrounding the globe, may be visible when the orbital septum has been lacerated. The orbital septum acts to separate the orbital contents from the more superficial muscles and the skin. Since the skin over the eyelids is extremely thin, any visible fat below the orbicularis oculi muscle is presumed to be periorbital fat. An immediate ophthalmologic consult and repair is needed. Likewise any laceration through the tarsal plate of the eyelid must be referred to an ophthalmologist for definitive care.

Deep lacerations to the medial half of the upper eyelid should be examined for a laceration to the tendon of the levator palpebrae superioris muscle. An injury to this tendon, which is deep to the orbicularis oculi muscle, may be evident by the patient's inability to lift the eyelid normally. A laceration or puncture to the medial one-fifth of the upper eyelid carries with it the potential for injury to the canaliculus of the lacrimal system. Any suspected injury to the lacrimal system requires an immediate ophthalmologic consult.

CHEEK LACERATIONS

Lacerations of the cheek may be repaired in the normal cosmetic fashion. However, the parotid duct and lacerated branches of the facial nerve (cranial nerve VII) must be repaired by a specialist.

The parotid (Stenson's) duct runs from the parotid gland along a line from the tragus of the ear to the mid-portion of the upper lip (Fig. 10.1). Parotid duct lacerations can be diagnosed by asking the patient to open the mouth wide in order to locate the punctate orifice of the duct. The orifice can be visualized on the buccal mucosa opposite the upper second premolar. Once located, the orifice is dried with gauze and the parotid gland is massaged. If clear fluid appears through the orifice, the duct can be considered intact. However, if no saliva or blood is expressed from the orifice, the duct should be considered injured or lacerated. A plastic surgery or ENT consult is required to evaluate the extent of the injury and initiate repair of the duct (as seen in Figure 10.2).

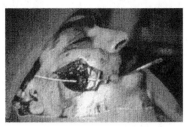

Figure 10.1 Cannulation of parotid duct after stab wound to cheek.

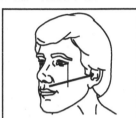

Figure 10.2 Landmarks for parotid duct and facial nerve location (see text).

The buccal and zygomatic branches of the facial nerve, which lie lateral to a vertical line dropped from the lateral canthus of the eye (Fig. 10.1), should be evaluated and repaired by a specialist when feasible. Failure to recognize and repair such nerve branches will affect the function of facial muscles of expression. Branches of the facial nerve medial to the vertical line generally are too fine and will not adversely affect muscle function.

NASAL WOUNDS

Nasal lacerations limited to the outer aspect of the nose should be repaired with 6-0 or 7-0 nylon or polypropylene and 5-0 or 6-0 vicryl or polydioxinone for muscle and dermal layers. Wounds to the cartilage should be closed in routine fashion after the cartilage has been placed in its proper anatomic position. Directly suturing the cartilage is not recommended as this may predispose the cartilage to infection and necrosis. Instead, the margins of the perichondrium should be apposed; thus bringing the cartilaginous edges together. Intranasal lacerations are best repaired by an ENT specialist. Minimal debridement of the cartilage should be performed only if absolutely necessary. Likewise, nasal skin should not be radically debrided because of the lack of redundant nasal tissue.

Examination of the nasal vestibule for a septal hematoma should always be performed. Septal hematomas are soft, fluctuant bulges of the nasal septal mucosa and are not ecchymotic. When such defects are not recognized and drained, necrosis and infection of the nasal cartilage can result. Perforation of the septum and/or a nasal deformity can ultimately result. Incision, drainage, nasal packing, and anti-staphylococcal antibiotic therapy is required after an ENT consult.

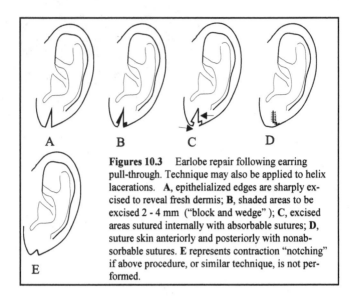

Figures 10.3 Earlobe repair following earring pull-through. Technique may also be applied to helix lacerations. **A**, epithelialized edges are sharply excised to reveal fresh dermis; **B**, shaded areas to be excised 2 - 4 mm ("block and wedge"); **C**, excised areas sutured internally with absorbable sutures; **D**, suture skin anteriorly and posteriorly with nonabsorbable sutures. **E** represents contraction "notching" if above procedure, or similar technique, is not performed.

Small, partial thickness avulsions, less than 1 cm², involving skin from the tip of the nose can be allowed to heal secondarily. Patients with larger or full-thickness avulsions to the nose should have an immediate plastic surgery consult or referral.

EAR WOUNDS

Lacerations to the helix of the ear that extend through the auricular cartilage and through-and-through lacerations to the lobe should be repaired using a "block and wedge cut" (Figs. 10.3 a-d) or a similar technique. This prevents notching of the ear due to contraction forces present on any semi-circular wound. As mentioned above, the cartilage should be apposed by suture placement in the perichondrium and/or dermis. Skin coverage is imperative to prevent desiccation, necrosis or infection of the cartilage due to its relatively poor blood supply.

If post-operative bleeding is anticipated, the ear should be wrapped with a conforming dressing. The convolutions of the ear are packed with saline-moistened, fluffed 2x2 gauze. The ear is then covered anteriorly and posteriorly with dry 4x4s and finally a circumferential head bandage. This dressing should remain undisturbed unless pain or wound infection is suspected. The patient should be instructed to return for a wound check in 24 - 48 hours.

Auricular hematomas or infections require surgical drainage. An anterior and /or posterior incision with a scalpel can be made in such a way that the resultant scar will be hidden from view. Following drainage, the wound should be dressed with a nonadhering gauze (i.e., xeroform) and an anatomically-conforming pressure dressing. The patient should be instructed to have the wound checked within 24 - 36 hours and should be placed on antibiotics. Serial drainage may be required to remove subsequent edema, prevent necrosis of the auricular cartilage and deformity formation, "cauliflower ear".

LIP WOUNDS

Lacerations that extend across the vermilion cutaneous border of the lip must be carefully and accurately repaired. Failure to be meticulous in alignment will result in an

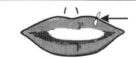

Figure 10.4 "Stay" suture placed at the vermilion cutaneous border of the lip before further repair is performed

unsatisfactory cosmetic result. To reduce further swelling of the lip and distortion of the wound margins at the vermilion border, an infraorbital or mental nerve block should be performed. However, very small wounds may be locally infiltrated or a field block can be performed. In addition, wound margin debridement at the vermilion border should be avoided whenever possible. Always examine the wound for broken tooth fragments and remove any fragments present.

For large, full-thickness lip wounds, the first step of repair involves the placement of a single nonabsorbable suture (6-0 nylon) exactly across the margins of the vermilion border (Fig 10.4). This is done to precisely appose the vermilion border margins and is often done after the orbicularis oris muscle has been reapproximated. The dermis and skin should then be sutured in the usual cosmetic fashion.

Small, partial-thickness wounds across the vermilion cutaneous border should be repaired only after the vermilion border is properly aligned.

Lacerations to the red tissue of the lip may be closed with either 6-0 fast-absorbing plain gut, vicryl *RAPIDE*® or soft polyester sutures. These sutures are more comfortable for the patient and the former two types of material do not require suture removal.

Deep lacerations of the lip, those extending into and through the orbicularis oris muscle into the oral cavity, should be repaired in layers to prevent retraction of the muscle and subsequent scar depression. The muscle is closed first with 5-0 absorbable suture such as vicryl or polydioxinone. The skin above the vermilion cutaneous border can be closed with 6-0 non-absorbable sutures while the red tissue of the lip can be repaired with 6-0 fast-absorbing plain gut. The intraoral component of a through-and-through lip laceration may be left unsutured if it is: 1) linear and less than 1 cm in length and 2) does not interfere with chewing or is not gaping. Small intraoral lacerations heal quickly with few complications. However, large intraoral lacerations that are non-linear or are likely to entrap food particles should be sutured last with absorbable sutures. Suturing the intraoral last lessens the risk of contaminating the instruments and healthy tissue than vice versa.

Skin avulsions of the lip and philtrum should be addressed by a plastic surgeon for cosmetic reasons.

"Swish and spit" rinses of half-strength hydrogen peroxide solution are recommended to promote healing and keep the mucosal surface "clean". Rinses can be used 5 - 6 times a day. Simple, non-communicating lacerations generally do not require antibiotics if a thorough wound prep is done. Patients with large or through-and-through lip lacerations should be covered with oral penicillin, clindamycin or erythromycin for 3 - 5 days. Application of cool compresses, or ice packs, is also recommended to reduce localized bleeding and edema.

TONGUE LACERATIONS

Small tongue lacerations and puncture wounds to the tongue do not require sutures. They will heal remarkably well without surgical intervention. The patient should be instructed to rinse or swab the tongue wound several times a day with a half-strength hydrogen peroxide solution.

Larger tongue lacerations should be sutured using absorbable material (i.e., 4-0, 5-0 vicryl, chromic gut, or vicryl *RAPIDE*®). Burying the knots, whenever possible, is preferable to having an exposed suture and its knot irritate the patient. Repairing the tongue often requires the assistance of another person to hold the tongue steady. The tongue may be held securely with gauze or a holding suture may be placed through the tip of the tongue and retracted by the assistant to facilitate repair. Conscious sedation may be helpful to repair such lacerations in very young, uncooperative children. Each institution's protocols for conscious sedation should be consulted and followed. Remember that even though the patient is sedated they are conscious and will still sense pain unless locally anesthetized. Always anesthetize the wound before repair.

"TRAP-DOOR DEFORMITY" of the FOREHEAD

Crescent or U-shaped lacerations to the forehead are often the result of persons being thrown into an automobile windshield, a sun visor, a rearview mirror, or striking the head on some sharp object. This type of injury poses a few management problems.

First, the edges of such wounds are almost always beveled or oblique. Ideally, the wound margins should be made perpendicular to the skin surface with minimal debridement, or excision, prior to closure. Second, as the

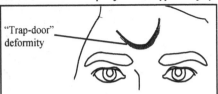

Figure 10.5 "Trap-door" deformity of the forehead. Note the shadow on inferior margin resulting from contraction and bulging of the flap. See text for possible preventive measures.

wound heals, contraction forces on the wound pull the wound margins toward the center of this crescent-shaped flap. Secondary intention healing or improper wound repair can result in the formation of a bulging scar or "trap-door" deformity weeks or months later (Fig. 10.5). Well-placed "anchoring" sutures can be used to attach and secure the center portion of the flap to the underlying tissues. "Anchoring" sutures are meant to prevent significant movement of the flap by wound contraction forces and to eliminate any dead spaces. Third, care must be taken to appose the severed frontalis muscle, when involved, to prevent a muscle retraction defect or impaired muscle function in the affected area. Finally, a firm but not too tight head dressing should be applied after the repair to prevent the formation of a hematoma. The dressing should be kept in place for about 4 days except for daily wound cleaning by the patient.

Despite even the most meticulous efforts, "trap-door" deformities can develop and may require wound revision if aesthetically unattractive.

SCALP LACERATIONS

When presented with deep lacerations to the scalp, the healthcare provider must look for more extensive underlying injuries. Skull fractures should be ruled out either by mechanism of injury and digital palpation with sterile gloves or by head CT. Caution should be exercised to ascertain the presence of foreign bodies, particularly sharp ones, prior to placing a gloved finger into the wound. Remove any foreign bodies found in the wound. Furthermore, one should never push on the skull but should gently feel for a bony depression or "step-off". If no bony abnormality is found, the galea and muscles should be sutured, followed by the skin. Repair of the skin in patients with dark hair is easier to accomplish with blue polypropylene sutures. As discussed in Section 7, scalp hair does not need to be shaved. Do not shave hairline margins as proper landmarks will be lost during repair. Blood clots and foreign bodies should be removed during the wound prep and before closure.

Occasionally, lacerations to small scalp arteries will be encountered. The administration of an anesthetic with epinephrine can be used to decrease, or even stop, bleeding. In some instances though, isolation and ligation of the small artery is required before suturing the wound. The two ends of the artery may be ligated with 5-0 plain or chromic gut. Alternatively, figure-of-eight sutures may be placed in the tissue around the retracted artery end to provide hemostasis.

Multiple abrasions or puncture wounds to the frontal scalp, usually from vehicle's occupant striking the windshield, must have each wound meticulously examined for pieces of glass or other foreign material. These wounds are often dismissed as simple abrasions but may harbor foreign bodies. Failure to recognize and remove foreign bodies will result in discomfort, disfiguring scars and the need to have the material removed at a later time.

UPPER EXTREMITY WOUNDS

Probably the most common crush injury seen in the emergency department is a finger or hand that has been caught in a car or house door. The resulting injury may be a painful contusion and subungual hematoma, a laceration, an open fracture, or a combination of these.

A **subungual hematoma,** or the accumulation of blood under the nail plate, can be treated in a simple and painless manner; affording the patient almost immediate relief from the pressure and throbbing. Before nail plate trephination (drainage), an x-ray should be obtained to rule out a fracture. Theoretically, trephination of a nail plate with an underlying fracture is tantamount to converting a closed fracture to an open fracture. Patients with open fractures should receive antibiotic prophylaxis.

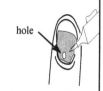

Figure 10.6 Evacuation of a subungual hematoma by nail plate trephination with cautery.

Hematomas may be trephinated if they are painful and/or less than 50% of the nail plate surface. Acute subungual hematomas comprising more than 50% of the nail plate surface should have the nail plate removed. Likewise, those which are less than 8 hours old and have a significant distal phalanx fracture should have the nail plate removed and the nail bed laceration repaired.

To trephinate a nail plate, one may use a heated paper clip, a large-bore needle or a battery-powered, fine-tipped cautery (pen-type). The latter is the

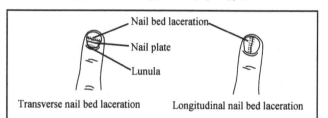

Transverse nail bed laceration   Longitudinal nail bed laceration

Figure 10.7 Nail bed laceration repairs requiring partial or complete nail plate removal.

easiest to handle and causes less discomfort (nail plate pressure) if used properly. The hematoma acts as a cushion between the nail plate and the sensitive nail bed. The tip of the device should go only through the nail plate (Fig. 10.6) and should not touch the nail bed. It should be withdrawn quickly once blood comes through the nail plate. In most cases, nerve block anesthesia need not be administered.

Nail plate lacerations or avulsions often signify the presence of a **nail bed laceration.** Failure to treat such injuries appropriately, may result in possible nail bed or nail plate deformity. As always, an x-ray should be taken to rule out a fracture. If the nail plate is avulsed or lacerated and the injury is less than 8 hours old, a digital nerve block should be performed. Next, the nail plate should be at least partially removed to facilitate the repair of any nail bed laceration. Proximal nail plate avulsions or longitudinal nail plate lacerations require the removal of the entire nail plate as described below. Patients with transverse nail plate or nail bed lacerations need only have enough proximal nail plate removed to make repair easier (Fig 10.7). Nail bed lacerations are sutured, under digital tourniquet, with 6-0 vicryl. Don't forget to remove the tourniquet before bandaging!

Controversy has long existed regarding **nail plate replacement** after its removal and nail bed repair. Some believe that placement of the nail plate, foil, or gauze between the eponychium and the nail bed is necessary to prevent adhesions. Furthermore, they believe that failure to replace the nail plate will result in no nail plate growth or painful emergence of the nail plate. Having stated that viewpoint, it must be said that the nail plate (or any other material) does NOT need to be placed under the eponychium for the new nail plate to grow or grow normally. It is true that an adhesion does occur but the nail plate will emerge in about 60 - 90 days. Incidentally, any material placed under the nail fold will have to be removed at some point - usually with discomfort to the patient. The appearance of the new nail plate is not dependent on adhesions but rather upon the condition of the nail bed following injury. Accurate approximation of the nail bed with sutures will afford the best possible results. Replacement of the nail plate does afford temporary protection of the nail bed during healing as does a dressing or small splint.

Under digital tourniquet, **nail plate removal** is accomplished by introducing a pair of closed iris scissors under the distal nailplate. The points of the scissors MUST always be kept pointing toward the nail plate and away from the nail bed. The scissors are gradually advanced under the nail plate and gently opened to dissect the nail plate from the nail bed. When the nail plate is free from the nail bed, the nailfolds should be carefully dissected away from the nail plate. The nail plate is then removed.

Minimal to moderate bleeding from the nail bed after closure and tourniquet removal requires antibiotic ointment, a non-adhering gauze and a bulky dressing application. Some post-repair skin maceration and dressing adherence can be expected. These conditions may be kept to a minimum if the dressing is changed in 24 hours and the hand is kept elevated above heart level. Any dressing that adheres after 24 hours may be soaked off with hydrogen peroxide. Dressings should be changed at least daily. Padded aluminum and "stack" finger splints are helpful in protecting the fingertip from further trauma until the nail grows back.

Skin avulsions can be treated simply with either an absorbable hemostat (i.e., gelfoam) or a non-adhering gauze (i.e., adaptic, xeroform) pressure dressing. Partial and full-thickness skin avulsions of less than 1 cm^2 will granulate and contract to less than one-third their original size - often with no decreased tactile function. Incomplete epidermal or thin split-thickness avulsions with a small pedicle can be debrided and allowed to heal by secondary intention. Elevation of the affected extremity for at least 24 hours will help reduce bleeding through the pressure dressing. Larger avulsions may be repaired, when possible, by excision of the wound margins, extension and undermining. Alternatively, if the avulsion is too large or does not lend itself to excision and undermining (i.e., the fingers), a

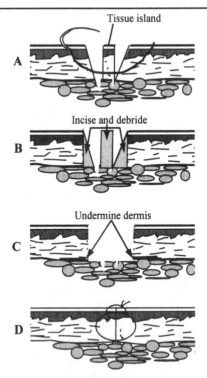

Figures 10.8 A-D. Tissue island repair - two techniques.
First technique: A, simple suturing of wound through tissue island with bite through same tissue level.
Second technique: B, perpendicular incisions on both wound margins to subcutaneous fat only with shaded areas showing tissue to be removed; **C**, excision and debridement of tissue island and undermining of tissue along dermal-subcutaneous fat border; and **D**, closure of the skin and dermis with sutures.

plastic surgery referral is warranted.

Webspace lacerations, particularly to the thenar webspace, pose a two-fold problem. First, there is a tendency for the skin to invert upon itself. Eversion of the wound margins is necessary for proper wound healing. This problem can be overcome by using a horizontal or vertical mattress suture or by the careful placement of a simple interrupted suture. Second, there is potential for development of dead space in the redundant webspace tissues for fluids to accumulate. This can lead to infection or other complications. After suturing, a slight compression dressing is helpful in reducing any dead space.

Puncture wounds to the hand or extremity, like most puncture wounds,

Principles of Primary Wound Management

should not be sutured unless the exact tissue depth can be determined. The mechanism of such an injury should be fully investigated. Punctures or small wounds appearing over the dorsum of the hand at the metacarpophalangeal (MCP) joints should be thought of as a human bite until proven otherwise. Such highly suspicious wounds should not be sutured as they will heal well by secondary intention. Antibiotics should be given to reduce the risk of infection. An x-ray should be taken to rule out a fracture but also the presence of a foreign body (i.e., broken tooth) or air in the joint.

Wounds with **tissue islands** pose a special management problem. These wounds result from contact with sharp objects such as escalator steps or a knife used by the suicidal patient to make multiple slash incisions. They appear as parallel wounds with very little space between each wound margin. Attempts to suture all of these wounds together is sometimes difficult or impossible. Suturing often results in the inversion of one or more of these tissue islands. Suture bites through the same tissue layer or excision of the tissue island(s) may make for a simpler repair and a more cosmetically-appealing scar (Fig 10.8).

A wound resulting from a **high pressure injection** gun is a true hand emergency and must be treated aggressively. The wound may appear small and innocuous on the surface but deep tissue damage occurs due to widespread contamination of injected grease, paint, or solvents. The injected substance often travels into tendon sheaths and dissects through fascial planes; following the path of least resistance. The morbidity is high when high pressure injection injuries are not recognized by history and examination and treated rapidly. X-rays are sometimes helpful in evaluating the extent of the injury when radiopaque substances have been injected. In any case, an immediate hand specialty consult is necessary to surgically debride the tissues and initiate antibiotic therapy.

LOWER EXTREMITY WOUNDS

Although almost any of the injuries discussed in the *Upper Extremity Wounds* subsection can be seen in the lower extremity, injuries unique to the lower extremities will be discussed here.

Pre-tibial lacerations, especially flap lacerations, should be treated conservatively. The mechanism of injury, the poor vascularity of the area, and the desire to leave the leg in a dependent position all predispose such wounds to lengthy healing processes. Closure without tension is necessary otherwise the viability of the flap is in jeopardy. As discussed on page 16, viability of flap lacerations on the extremities is always a concern due to venous congestion and post-injury edema. To increase the likelihood of flap survival, one may suture one flap margin with a minimum of sutures and allow the other margin to be held in position with steri-strips while granulation takes place. This is particularly helpful for patients with atrophic (thin) skin lacerations. Small flaps may be excised and converted into linear wounds. All patients should be instructed to keep the extremity elevated above heart level for 48 - 72 hours to reduce edema and promote drainage from the flap.

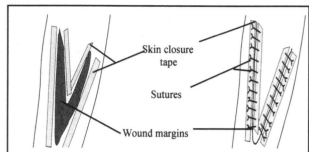

Figure 10.9 Alternative method for the repair of atrophic ("thin-skin") lacerations utilizing skin closure tape (i.e., Proxi-Strip, Steri-strip) to reinforce wound margins and prevent pull-throughs.

Knee lacerations should be closed with simple interrupted sutures, mattress sutures, or a combination of these two techniques. Knee lacerations, with the exception of small or superficial wounds, usually require intradermal sutures to keep the wound margins tension-free during healing. Patients with such wounds should also have a knee immobilizer applied to restrict flexion and extension of the knee. The immobilizer should be kept on for no more than seven days, excluding time for dressing changes and short passive exercise sessions. The immobilization time may vary from person to person and upon the severity of the injury.

ATROPHIC SKIN WOUNDS

An alternative method of treatment for atrophic skin lacerations mentioned above involves the application of skin closure tape (i.e., Proxi-Strip, Steri-strip) on both the flap and non-flap wound margins (Fig. 10.9). Do not use tincture of benzoin on the skin before applying the skin closure tape. Once the skin closure tape (Proxi-Strips, Steri-strip) is applied, the wound may be sutured with each suture bite passing through the tape. This method of reinforcing the edges often prevents tearing of the thin wound edges and improves the chance of healing.

PRESERVATION OF AMPUTATED DIGITS

Amputated appendages (i.e., fingers, toes, ears, nose, penis) should be transported and handled carefully to preserve tissue integrity and improve replantation success. All amputated body parts should be rinsed of any gross contamination before being placed in a sterile, saline-moistened gauze or cloth. Immersion of the body part directly in saline or water jeopardizes the salvagability of the tissue. Likewise, no sharp excision or debridement should be performed except by the specialist. The gauze and body part should then be placed into a sealed plastic bag and placed in a container of ice-water. Ice should be replaced as necessary. Dry ice should NEVER be used to preserve tissue.

Replantation criteria includes the general health and age of the patient, the mechanism of injury, the amount of tissue damage, the time lapse from injury to repair, and the method and temperature of preservation of the amputated part. The replantation specialist must make the ultimate decision whether to use or discard the tissue.

MISCELLANEOUS SURGICAL PROCEDURES

FOREIGN BODY REMOVAL

The first step in the removal of any foreign body is to determine the size and the location of the object. This may be done by palpation of the object under the skin or it may require radiographic studies. As always, assess the neuro-motor-vascular status prior to proceeding with removal of the foreign body.

SIMPLE FOREIGN BODY REMOVAL (i.e., wooden sliver under nail plate)

1   Administer local or peripheral nerve block anesthesia.
2   Prep skin with povidone-iodine solution.
3   Remove the object with forceps or hemostats (sometimes a wedge of nail plate needs to be removed).
4   Irrigate the wound tract with normal saline under pressure.
5   Dress the wound.
6   Consider antibiotic if cellulitis is present.

COMPLICATED REMOVAL (unseen foreign body; i.e., needle or wood in the foot)

1   X-ray the area with a marker taped over or to the side of the entry point. If the foreign body is too deep, refer patient to a specialist for possible removal in the operating room.
2   Administer local or peripheral nerve block anesthesia.
3   Prep the skin with povidone-iodine solution.
4   Apply tourniquet, where feasible, to provide a bloodless field.
5   Set a reasonable amount of time (20-30 minutes) to locate the foreign body. If unsuccessful after this allotted time, defer to a specialist.
6   Make an incision over the foreign body tract or whenever possible make an incision perpendicular to the foreign body tract.
7   Carefully use blunt dissection to locate and visualize the object.
8   Isolate the object and clamp only onto the foreign body with hemostats. Remember not to clamp in a bloody field and never clamp blindly - especially in the hand.
9   Remove the foreign body from the skin without unclamping the hemostats.
10 Clean and irrigate the wound tract with normal saline. Do not insert the catheter or needle into the tract.
11 The wound may be: sutured primarily, allowed to heal by secondary intention, or closed on a delayed basis. Check for small fragments before closing. If in doubt, leave it open.
12 Dress the wound appropriately.
13 Advise the patient to observe for signs of infection. Consider antibiotics.

"DOG EAR" REPAIR

A "dog ear" repair is actually a surgical way to correct a mistake in technique made during the wound repair. It is characterized by an excess of tissue at one end of the wound. This can be avoided by carefully matching each wound margin as one sutures. The illustrations (Fig. 11.1) show how one goes about performing the corrective procedure.

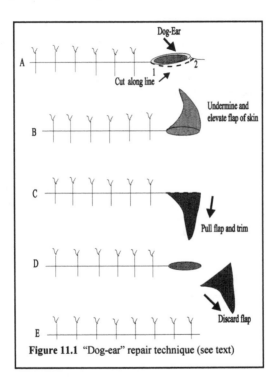

Figure 11.1 "Dog-ear" repair technique (see text)

DELAYED PRIMARY REPAIR

Delayed primary repair or closure (DPR) is a time-tested procedure to reduce the amount of healing time for old or contaminated wounds. In addition, the cosmetic appearance of the wound is much improved versus a wound allowed to heal by secondary intention. Wounds that qualify for a DPR are: open wounds in a cosmetically significant location that exhibit no signs of infection 4 - 6 days (96 - 144 hours) following injury. When considering a DPR, one must remember:

1   The wound is anesthetized and prepped in the normal fashion after a

thorough examination on Day 1.

2	All devitalized tissue and debris must be removed on Day 1.

3	The wound should not be sutured or taped but left open. The open wound should be packed with saline-soaked 4x4 non-cotton gauze sponges. The gauze must make contact with the wound margins and the depth of the wound to be effective. The intent is to have these sponges dry out over the next 4 - 6 days; thus creating a wet-to-dry dressing.

4	The patient should be instructed to leave the bandage undisturbed, unless it is believed an infection is developing.

5	In 4 - 6 days following the initial visit, the dressing is removed. When removed, the sponges will automatically debride the wound to some extent.

6	A good healing ridge of granulation tissue should be noticeable.

7	*DPR may only be performed if there are no signs of infection present.*

8	If the wound is healthy appearing, it may be anesthetized and prepped. If the wound appears infected, clean the wound and treat with antibiotics. Refer to surgeon for follow-up.

9	The wound edges are sharply excised with a #15 scalpel blade to remove the granulation tissue before suturing. Failure to remove this epithelialized tissue will result in non-union of the wound edges.

10	After excision, the wound is irrigated, sutured and dressed.

11	The patient should be asked to return within 48 hours for a wound check.

12	Sutures may be removed according to suggested guidelines.

COMMON ORTHOPEDIC INJURIES OF THE HAND

MALLET FINGER ("baseball finger")

Mallet finger is a relatively simple extensor tendon injury to recognize and treat primarily. It results from the traumatic avulsion of the terminal extensor tendon of the finger from the dorsal base of the distal phalanx (Fig. 12.1). This injury can be associated with or without a fracture of the base of the distal phalanx. Furthermore, it may be an open or a closed injury. Regardless, an x-ray is required prior to treatment.

The patient with a mallet finger presents with a flexed distal interphalangeal (DIP) joint in which there is complete passive but absent active extension of the DIP joint. Treatment consists of wearing a splint, with the DIP joint held in extension, continuously for 6-8 weeks; followed by another 2 weeks at nighttime. The splint can be applied either dorsally or volarly from the PIP joint to the tip of the finger; leaving the proximal interphalangeal joint free to flex and extend. Surgical wire fixation by a hand specialist may be necessary for some deformities for intratircular fractures of more than 25 percent. Hand specialist referral and follow-up is needed. The patient should be strongly advised not to remove the splint as this may adversely affect healing of this injury.

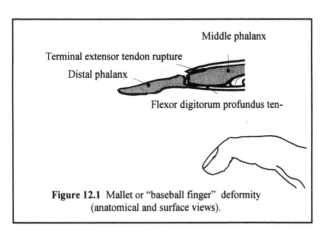

Middle phalanx

Terminal extensor tendon rupture

Distal phalanx

Flexor digitorum profundus ten-

Figure 12.1 Mallet or "baseball finger" deformity (anatomical and surface views).

BOUTONNIERE DEFORMITY

A **boutonniere deformity** is the result of a laceration or rupture of the central slip of the extensor tendon mechanism of the finger (Fig. 12.2). The lateral bands of the extensor tendon sublux volarly and become paradoxical flexors of the PIP joint. The extensor mechanism is shortened; thus hyperextending the DIP joint. Like the mallet finger injury, the boutonniere may be an open or closed injury. Treatment consists of the application of a splint to the dorsum of the finger with the PIP joint extended. Both the MCP and DIP joints are allowed full range of motion. The splint should remain undisturbed for at least 6 weeks unless removed by the hand specialist in follow-up.

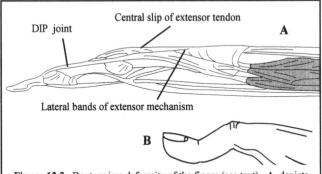

Figure 12.2 Boutonniere deformity of the finger (see text). **A**, depicts anatomical structure involved and **B** exhibits the external appearance of the digit with such a deformity.

GAMEKEEPER'S THUMB ("skier's thumb")

Gamekeeper's thumb is the partial or complete rupture of the ulnar collateral ligament of the thumb at the metacarpophalangeal (MCP) joint (Fig. 12.3). The injury gets its name from injuries suffered by Scottish gamekeepers after they killed rabbits and fowl by cervical dislocation. Today, it is commonly seen when skiers fall and get their thumbs entangled in the ski pole strap. This causes the thumb to subluxate radially, thereby weakening the pinch function of the thumb.

Examination of the injured thumb is carried out by flexing the IP and MCP joints of the thumb and radially subluxating the digit. An incomplete rupture is suspected if the joint is painful with subluxation but opens no more than 45 degrees. Treatment for an incomplete rupture is a thumb spica splint for 6 - 8 weeks and frequent assessment by an orthopedic surgeon. Complete rupture, or laxity of the ulnar collateral ligament more

Figure 12.2. Gamekeeper's (or skier's) thumb.

than 45° when the MCP joint is stressed, requires surgical repair and splinting.

SCAPHOID FRACTURES

Any patient presenting with a closed, painful wrist injury should be evaluated for a **scaphoid fracture**. The scaphoid is the most commonly fractured bone in the wrist. Fractures usually occur following a fall on an outstretched hand. A fracture through the waist (Fig. 12.4) or proximal pole of the scaphoid threatens the bone's distal blood supply; thus causing an avascular necrosis in

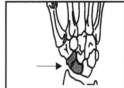

Figure 12.4 Fracture through the waist of the scaphoid.

the proximal fragment. Anatomical snuffbox tenderness warrants an x-ray, including a scaphoid view. Most of the time, however, fractures of the scaphoid are not detected by initial radiographic study. The patient should be treated on the clinical findings with thumb spica splint, referred to an orthopedic surgeon, and instructed to have a repeat x-ray in 2 weeks. This additional time is needed for the bone to reabsorb and reveal the fracture line on x-ray.

It is always better to overtreat, by immobilization with a thumb spica splint, any wrist injury with snuffbox tenderness rather than dismiss the injury as a sprained wrist and do nothing.

BOXER'S FRACTURE

A **boxer's fracture,** or a fracture of the fifth metacarpal, is usually sustained by punching a hard object (i.e., another person's face or a wall) with a closed fist (Fig. 12.5). These fractures, if not severely displaced, open, angulated, or rotated, should be immobilized in an ulnar gutter splint and referred to an orthopedic surgeon for follow-up. Open wounds over

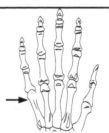

Figure 12.5 Boxer's fracture of the 5th metacarpal neck.

the joints should be cleaned and dressed but not sutured. If caused by striking teeth, the patient should be given the appropriate prophylactic antibiotic.

Dorsal angulation of the head of the metacarpal up to 40° is usually acceptable by the orthopedist. However, one must evaluate the patient for a rotational malalignment of the fingertip. This can be done by asking the patient to flex the MCP and PIP joints and assessing the alignment of the fingers; the tip should point to the scaphoid bone (Fig. 12.6).

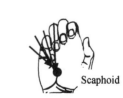

Figure 12.6 Assessment of rotational malalignment of the fingers (see text).

Overlapping or divergence of the fingertips needs an orthopedic referral.

one must evaluate the patient for a rotational malalignment of the fingertip. This can be done by asking the patient to flex the MCP and PIP joints and assessing the alignment of the fingers; the tip should point to the scaphoid bone (Fig. 12.6). Overlapping or divergence of the fingertips needs a hand or orthopedic referral for correction of any rotation.

ORTHOPEDIC SPLINTING

Post-injury splinting and immobilization hastens healing of injured tissues and prevents further injury or deformity. In most cases, the splint or device maintains a position of function; that is, a position that requires a minimum amount of rehabilitative time and/or joint stiffness following injury. Basic fracture or sprain principles include Protection, Rest, Ice, Compression, Elevation, and Support.

There are several different types of orthopedic splinting materials and devices commercially available. By far, plaster remains the most popular material for splinting and casting with fiberglass a close second. Both are available in rolls, sheets, and ready-to-use padded rolls.

When using plaster or fiberglass, the provider should refer to the following guidelines to achieve the best results.

* Make sure the width and length of the splint are correct for the patient.
* Make the thickness of the splint, if not already pre-made, suitable for its purpose. About 12 - 15 layers of plaster should be used for most adult splints. More layers or reinforcement may be needed for certain areas under stress. Fiberglass requires fewer layers of the material than does plaster.
* Apply adequate protection (i.e., cast underpadding) to the patient's skin prior to the application of the splint. This will reduce skin maceration and direct contact with the plaster or fiberglass. If ready-to-use roll material used, additional padding may not be needed.
* Always use fresh, cool water for wetting the plaster or fiberglass. Plaster-contaminated water and warm water permits the material to set up too quickly and produces a more exothermic reaction.
* Place the plaster or fiberglass on a flat surface and push all individual layers of the material together to make a solid slab. This will remove most air pockets and is called lamination.
* Ring out excess water. Use a towel if necessary to remove water from the ready-to-use roll covering.
* Secure the splint firmly to the extremity but not too tightly with ace wraps.
* Position the splint to the desired joint angles.
* Explain to the patient that there may be some heat felt during the curing of the plaster or fiberglass. Assure the patient that the heat will not increase to the point of burning or injuring them. It should only last for about 10 - 15 minutes. If the heat becomes a concern to the patient, unwrap and remove the drying splint, make the patient comfortable (cool the skin if necessary), and replace the splint may be reapplied once it is cool.

Be sure to ascertain and document the sensory and vascular status prior to and after splint application.

Described on the following pages are several splints for the treatment of upper and lower extremity injuries.

DORSAL HAND SPLINT (Figure 13.1)

Indications: Metacarpal fractures, proximal phalanx fractures, crush injuries and soft tissue injuries of the hand.

Splint angles: Wrist: 20° - 30° of extension
MCP joints: 70° - 90° of flexion
IP joints: 10° - 20° of flexion

Application:
- Place two opened 4x4 gauze pads between all fingers and pad the palm. The gauze help absorb perspiration between the finger thereby decreasing skin maceration. Helps hold the concavity of the palm when the hand is splinted.
- Apply 3 - 5 inch wide splint material to the dorsum of the hand from the mid-forearm to the distal nailplate with the angles above.
- Leave the nailplates exposed to check capillary refill.
- Secure the splint with 2 inch ace wrap or roll gauze. Make sure it is not too tight or loose.

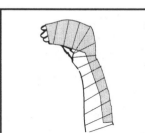

Figure 13.1 Dorsal hand splint.

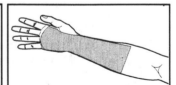

Figure 13.2 Volar wrist splint before ace wrap application.. Note that the MCP joints and thumb are not incorporated in the splint.

VOLAR WRIST SPLINT (Figure 13.2)

Indications: Wrist sprains, carpal fractures, non-displaced radius and ulnar styloid fractures, and carpal tunnel syndrome.

Splint angle: Wrist: 20° - 30° of extension

Application: Apply 3 - 5 inch wide splint material to the volar surface of the forearm from the mid-forearm to the MCP joint creases. Set wrist angle as above.

- The MCP joints should retain full flexion and extension.
- Secure the splint with 2 inch ace wrap or roll gauze. Make sure the fit it is not too tight or too loose.

SUGAR TONG (STIRRUP) SPLINT of the FOREARM (Figure 13.3)

Indications: Fractures of the radius and ulna

Splint angles: Wrist: 20° - 30° of extension
                   Elbow: 90° of flexion

Application:
- Apply 3 - 5 inch wide splint material to the volar aspect of the hand and forearm, beginning proximal to the MCP joint creases.
- Extend material from the wrist around the elbow to the dorsum of the forearm and stop at the dorsal MCP joints.
- Set angles as above.
- Secure the splint with 3 or 4 inch ace wraps or roll gauze.
- Apply arm sling to carry the weight of the splint.
- Do not extend the splint beyond the MCP joints. There should be full flexion and extension of the joints.

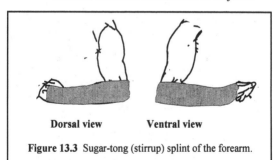

Dorsal view   **Ventral view**

Figure 13.3 Sugar-tong (stirrup) splint of the forearm.

POSTERIOR SPLINT of the ELBOW (Figure 13.4)

Indications: Fractures of the radius and ulna, elbow, post-reduction of elbow dislocations, soft tissue injuries of the elbow, distal humerus fractures.

Splint angles: Wrist: 20° - 30° of extension
                   Elbow: 90° of flexion

Application:

- Apply 3 - 5 inch wide splint material to the ulnar aspect of the arm, from mid-palm to mid-humerus, at the angles above.
- DO NOT incorporate the MCP joints.
- Secure the splint with 3 or 4 inch ace wraps or roll gauze.
- Apply arm sling to carry the weight of the splint.

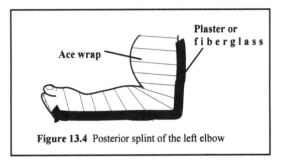

Plaster or fiberglass

Ace wrap

Figure 13.4 Posterior splint of the left elbow

THUMB SPICA SPLINT (Figure 13.5)

Indications: Crush injuries, fractures or dislocations of the thumb, and thenar contusions, scaphoid fractures, and gamekeeper's thumb should have a thumb spica splint.

Splint angles:
Wrist:	$20°$ - $30°$ of extension
Thumb:	- abducted $60°$ - $80°$ for a spica splint
	- slight ulnar deviation to relax ulnar collateral ligament in gamekeeper's thumb

Application:

- Apply 3 - 5 inch wide splint material from the mid-forearm to the thumb along the radial aspect of the thumb, at the desired angles indicated above.
- The thumb should be almost entirely incorporated into the splint. Do leave the tips visible to check capillary refill.
- Secure the splint with 2 or 3 inch ace wrap or roll gauze.

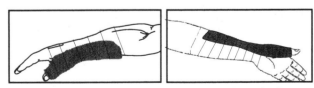

Figure 13.5 Thumb spica splint (dorsal and palmar views)

ULNAR GUTTER SPLINT (Figure 13.6)

Indications: Boxer's fractures, injuries to the ring and little fingers, hypothenar eminence, soft tissue or isolated bony injuries to the ulnar styloid.

Splint angles: Wrist: 20° - 30° of extension
                   MCP joints: 70° - 90° of flexion
                   IP joints: 10° - 20° of flexion

Application:
- Apply 3 - 5 inch wide splint material along the ulnar aspect of the mid-forearm to the DIP joints of the ring and little fingers, at the angles indicated above.
- Secure the splint with 2 inch ace wrap or roll gauze.

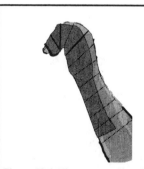

Figure 13.6 Ulnar gutter splint of the wrist.

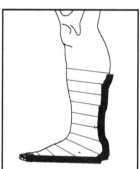

Figure 13.7 Posterior ankle splint.

POSTERIOR SPLINT of the ANKLE (Figure 13.7)

Indications: Ankle sprains, nondisplaced ankle fractures, metatarsal fractures, soft tissue injuries of the foot and ankle.

Splint angles: Ankle: 90°   (neutral or right angle position)
                   45° - 60°   plantar flexion (Achilles tendon ruptures)

Application:
- Apply 4 - 6 inch wide splint material from the toes along the plantar surface of the foot extending to the posterior aspect of the ankle, ending approximately halfway up the posterior calf.
- Secure the splint with two 4-inch ace wraps or roll gauze.
- This splint is not designed for weight-bearing. Patient must use crutches.

SUGAR TONG (STIRRUP) of the ANKLE (Figure 13.8)

Indications: Excellent for inversion / eversion ankle sprains and
                 nondisplaced ankle fractures

Splint angles: Ankle: 90°   (neutral or right angle position)

Application:
- Apply 4 - 6 inch wide splint material from the lateral
  aspect of the mid-lower leg around the heel to the medial
  aspect of the mid-lower leg.
- Secure the splint with two 4-inch ace wraps or roll gauze.
- This splint is not designed for weight-bearing. Patient
  must use crutches.

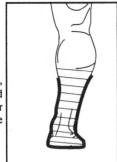

Note: There are also pre-formed splints (i.e.,
Air-Stirrup®) which can be applied and removed
with Velcro fasteners and provide support for
inversion / eversion ankle sprains. They may be
worn inside a sneaker for support when walking.

Figure 13.8 Sugar
tong (stirrup) ankle

ALUMINUM DIGITAL SPLINT

Indications: Finger contusions or sprains, distal tuft fractures, non-
                 displaced phalanx fractures, digital dislocations, and
                 tendon injuries such as mallet finger, boutonniere
                 deformity.

Splint angles: Varies according to injury and purpose; from protection to
                 position of function.

Application: Obtain desired length or cut to fit. Mold to desired
                 shape and angles. Tape in place with foam padding
                 toward the finger. May be taped to either the dorsum or
                 volar surface of the digit.

Following the application of any of the splints described above or any
immobilization device, one must check and observe for signs of poor
circulation. The most common signs are: tissue cyanosis, poor capillary

refill, increasing pain, loss of sensation distal to the injury, paresthesias, and cool tissue temperature.

Basic Splint Care Instructions for the Patient

First and foremost, instruct the patient to keep the splint dry. Splint material is not waterproof and plaster is not designed to maintain its strength and form when wet. If the splint can be removed (i.e., mild sprains), instruct the patient to carefully remove it, wash and dry the skin thoroughly, then reapply the splint. If the splint should not be removed for several days, instruct the patient to either sponge bathe, bathe with the extremity out of the water, or use a plastic bag to keep the splint dry.

When applying splints, the ace wrap or roll gauze should not be too tight or too loose - it should only hold the splint firmly in place. Have the patient check sensory distal to the splint.

Lower extremity splints are not designed to withstand the patient's weight. Posterior ankle splints, in particular, will break just above the heel; rendering the splint useless. Instruct the patient to use crutches.

Advise the patient that prolonged immobility will result in joint stiffness and longer recovery times. Whenever indicated, suggest early mobilization.

MISCELLANEOUS ORTHOPEDIC DEVICES

This section will briefly discuss the indications and correct procedures for the application of various commonly used orthopedic devices.

Ace bandages are used for compression to control swelling following injury. They should be applied in a distal to proximal fashion, continuously overlapping about one-half the width of the previous underlying layer. For example, when applying ace bandages to the ankle, one should remember to incorporate the entire heel in the wrap. Some providers are accustomed to not including the heel; thereby, creating an area where edema can settle. Cast underpadding may be applied under the ace bandage to provide a little more support, compression, and comfort.

"Buddy-taping" is indicated for a variety of minor orthopedic injuries: contused fingers and toes, immobilization of reduced finger or toe dislocations, or small fractures of the phalanges. When "buddy taping" the digits, one must remember to place an absorbent piece of cotton, cast underpadding or 2x2 gauze between the digits to lessen maceration. The tape is applied for support but not tightly.

Rehabilitative **knee immobilizers** are used to keep the knee joint protected and stationary following trauma such as knee lacerations, effusions, ligamentous injuries, or significant contusions. The knee is kept slightly flexed at about 15 degrees. They may be used either under or over clothing and removed, depending upon the injury, for wound cleaning and passive movement.

Arm slings styles vary from simple triangular bandages to heavy cloth with Velcro fasteners. They are simply used to keep the upper extremity motion-restricted, treat clavicle fractures, or to help support the weight of a cast or splint. One must remember to properly fit the sling to the patient. All to often the patient's entire hand and wrist are seen outside the sling - this is incorrect. The sling should extend past the wrist and up to the MCP joints. This simple effort will prevent undue pressure and neurapraxia of the cutaneous branches of the ulnar nerve at the wrist.

The **sling and swathe**, or shoulder immobilizer, comes in many styles but is designed to restrict motion of the entire upper extremity, including the shoulder. It is primarily indicated following the reduction of shoulder dislocations and humerus fractures. Application is similar to that of the simple arm sling, except that there is an additional piece of fabric (or fastening strap) which is positioned around the back of the patient and attaches to the sling portion.

COMMON SOFT TISSUE INFECTIONS

This discussion of soft tissue infections will focus on the recognition and treatment of common infections of the hand, the treatment of small soft tissue abscesses, and tetanus and rabies immunization schedules.

PARONYCHIA

A **paronychia** is an infection of the soft tissue around the nail plate. It may be caused by the introduction of bacteria or chemicals under the paronychium, nail biting or a "hangnail". The predominant pathogen is staphylococcus. This infection presents with erythema, swelling, pus, and tenderness around the nail plate. It may be incised and drained with a #11 scalpel blade following a digital nerve block to make the patient more comfortable and cooperative. A small incision is made parallel to the nail plate into the nail fold at the site of greatest fluctuance (Fig. 14.1). The patient is advised to soak the affected digit in warm water 4 - 5 times a day for the first 2 days, change the bandage several times a day, keep the hand elevated for 24 - 48 hours, and return if the infection returns or worsens. Paronychias with ascending lymphangitis or cellulitis require antibiotics; otherwise these are localized infections treated surgically.

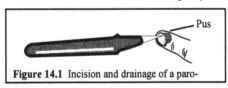

Figure 14.1 Incision and drainage of a paro-

SUBUNGUAL ABSCESS

Infections that extend underneath the nail plate are called **subungual abscesses**. Such infection may result from the presence or decay of a foreign body under the nail plate or a paronychia that has seeded the area under the nail plate. In any case, the nail plate should be removed and the nail bed cleaned and irrigated with normal saline. Trephination of the nail plate in an attempt to drain all of the pus from beneath the nail plate does not yield satisfactory results. Failure to eliminate all purulent material causes erosion and deformity of the nail bed. Once the nail plate has been removed and the area cleaned, antibiotics are usually not necessary unless there is an associated cellulitis. The patient may be discharged home with instructions to change the dressing frequently, wash the area with soap and water and return if problems develop.

FELON

A **felon** is an infection of the volar pulp space of the distal phalanx. It presents as an edematous, erythematous, and very tender distal phalanx and volar fat pad. The infection is confined to the pulp space by fibrous septae.

Felons should be incised longitudinally and drained where pointing, usually on the fat pad (Fig. 14.2). Care must be taken not to make an incision on the "pinch" side of any finger (i.e., radial border of index finger) since this will cause a sensitive scar. Transverse incisions, across the volar fat pad, are likely to transect the neuro-vascular bundle; therefore, these incisions are to be avoided. Likewise, the old-fashioned "fishmouth" or

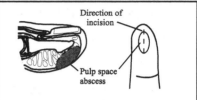

Figure 14.2 Location of fingertip felon and direction of required incision for drainage (see text).

"hockey- stick" incisions are not recommended as these tend to injure too much tissue at the tip of the digit; resulting in more of a deformity. Antibiotic therapy should be initiated on all patients with felons.

FLEXOR TENOSYNOVITIS

Flexor tenosynovitis, an infection of the flexor tendon sheath, is a hand emergency requiring hospital admission for antibiotic therapy and surgical drainage by a hand surgeon. Flexor tenosynovitis is characterized by Kanavel's four cardinal signs: 1) pain on passive extension of the digit, 2) the finger is held in a slightly flexed position, 3) there is uniform swelling of the digit, and 4) there is tenderness along the flexor tendon sheath.

After consultation with a hand surgeon, some early cases may be treated with intravenous antibiotics only and careful observation for progression of infection. Surgical intervention is needed for established cases to remove purulent material and prevent destruction of the tendons, sheaths, and development of adhesions between the tendons and the sheaths. These adhesions will adversely affect the smooth gliding ability of the tendons in the sheaths; thus interfering with flexion of the fingers.

SOFT TISSUE ABSCESSES

Fluctuant abscesses are simply treated by incision and drainage, followed by wick (drain) insertion, and bulky dressing application. Abscesses that present indurated (erythematous and firm without an area of fluctuance) may not be incised and drained initially because little, if any, pus will be expressed. Instead, the patient should be instructed to apply warm compresses several times a day to the area and seek surgical follow-up in about 72 hours for re-evaluation and possible incision. Alternatively,

Sitz baths are helpful for early perirectal abscesses, abscesses around the buttocks or following incision and drainage of abscesses in those areas. Antibiotics may be used for several days by some providers to eliminate the infection and need for surgical intervention. Certainly if fever develops, follow-up should be sought earlier.

The steps for simple skin abscess drainage are:

1   Make the patient as comfortable as possible.
2   X-ray if a foreign body is suspected (i.e., broken IV drug needle).
3   Use a local anesthetic by local infiltration or field block. Systemic drugs (i.e., intravenous midazolam) should be considered and given for larger abscesses, followed by a local anesthetic. Use care when infiltrating into the abscess as the needle may track the infection to healthy tissue.
4   Prepare the skin with povidone-iodine solution.
5   Using sterile technique, make a single incision with a #11 scalpel blade into the area of greatest fluctuance. Make the incision large enough to have pus flow freely from the abscess. Care should be taken not to go too deep - know the underlying anatomy before the incision and drainage is performed.
6   Express as much pus as possible by gentle digital manipulation and then use hemostats to break up the loculated pus.
7   Consider normal saline irrigation of the abscess before placing wick. Do not insert catheter into abscess while irrigating as this may seed healthy tissue.
8   Loosely insert an wick (plain or iodoform ribbon packing gauze) into the cavity to facilitate drainage and prevent reformation of the abscess.
9   Dress the abscess site with 4x4s and secure.

TETANUS

Tetanus-prone wounds are: puncture wounds, crush injuries, burns, frostbite, wounds over 6 hours old, stellate wounds, wounds greater than 1cm long, wounds with devitalized tissue, and wounds with organic contamination present.

Non-tetanus prone wounds are: wounds under 6 hours old, wounds with linear margins less than 1 cm long with no devitalized tissue or organic contamination, and wounds caused by sharp surfaces (knife, glass, metal).

The table on page 93 explains the anti-tetanus prophylaxis immunization schedule according to the Centers for Disease Control and Prevention (*MMWR* 39:37, 1990; MMWR 46(SS-2):15, 1997).

History of Tetanus	Tetanus-Prone Wound		Non-Tetanus Prone Wound	
	Td [1]	TIG [2]	Td [1]	TIG [2]
Unknown, > 25 yrs ago, or < 3 doses	YES	YES	YES	NO
3 or more doses with last > 5 years ago	YES	NO	YES [3]	NO
3 or more doses with last < 5 years ago	NO	NO	NO	NO

[1] Td = Tetanus and diphtheria toxoid adsorbed (adult) 0.5 cc IM
DPT in children less than 7 years old

[2] TIG = Tetanus immune globulin (human) 250 - 500 units IM

[3] = Yes if more than 10 years since last booster

RABIES

Rabies remains a threat to humans worldwide, especially in under-developed countries. Rabies post-exposure prophylaxis should be started   following immediate and thorough wound cleansing.

Any unprovoked attack or contact with suspected rabid mammals such as skunks, raccoons, bats, foxes, dogs, cats, or most carnivores should prompt immediate vaccination. Rabies is rarely seen in rodents, rabbits, voles, moles, squirrels, hamsters, guinea pigs, gerbils, chipmunks, and livestock but each case must be considered individually. If in doubt, contact your local public health officials and/or animal control authorities. Incubation ranges from 5 days to over 1 year with one reported case as long as 19 years.

Rabies post-exposure prophylaxis guidelines for *unvaccinated* persons as set forth by the Centers for Disease Control and Prevention (*MMWR* 48: RR-1, 1998; CID 30:4, 2000*)* consists of:

1) Human rabies immune globulin at 20 IU / kilogram body weight, with ½ of the dose injected around the wound (s) when anatomically feasible and the other ½ injected IM gluteal region is given ONCE on day 0
and

2) Human diploid cell vaccine (RabAvert® or Imovax®) 1.0 ml injected IM in the deltoid in adults and older children. Infants and young children should receive the injection in the anterolateral (outer) thigh. The HDCV is given on days 0, 3, 7, 14, and 28. *The HDCV should never be administered in the gluteal area for either group of patients or in the same syringe as the RIG (human).*

Previously vaccinated persons, according to the schedule above, who suspect or have a known contact with a rabid animal should receive only 2 doses of the HDCV; 1.0 ml IM deltoid on days 0 and 3. They should not receive HRIG if previously vaccinated.

BURNS

Burns are responsible for injuring more than two million people per year in the United States. More than 100,000 people annually require hospitalization for severe burns. An estimated 20,000 deaths per year are attributable to burns.

Burns, whether thermal, chemical, or electrical, cannot only be disfiguring but also account for a great amount of lost work time and normal daily activity. This discussion will be limited to so-called minor and moderate burns and will discuss the treatment modalities for each. The criteria for major burn classification and burn center transfer criteria will also be outlined. However, major burn treatment protocols will not be discussed since it beyond the scope of this text. Patients with severe or extensive burns should be transferred to the closest burn center.

BURN MECHANISMS

Thermal burns may be caused by moist heat, such as steam, boiling water or greases. In addition, they may be the result of dry heat, such as flames or hot metals.

Chemical burns are the result of exposure of the skin to acids (i.e., sulfuric, nitric, hydrofluoric acids) or alkalines (i.e., lye, cement, plaster, sodium hydroxide, bleach). Alkaline burns are more serious because of their ability to penetrate tissues quickly, denature proteins rapidly, and are difficult to irrigate out.

Electrical burns can be caused by the arcing of an electrical power source and a person's body - flash burns. Another cause of electrical burns is lightning or conductive injuries. The severity of the injury depends upon

Table 15.1 Burn Severity Classification (American Burn Association)

BURN SEVERITY	SECOND DEGREE	THIRD DEGREE
CRITICAL	Burns associated with inhalation injury and/ or fractures. Burns >30 % TBSA.	Burns associated with inhalation injury and / or fractures. Burns >10% TBSA. Burns of the face,
MODERATE	Burns involving 15 - 30 % TBSA.	Burns involving 2 - 10% TBSA and NOT involving the hands,
MINOR	Burns less than 15 % TBSA	Burns less than 2 % TBSA.

Table 15.2 Lund and Browder chart (percent total body surface area, % TBSA, by anatomical location and patient age)

Anatomical Location	Age (in years)				
Neck	2	2	2	2	2
Head	19	17	13	10	7
Anterior Trunk	13	13	13	13	13
Posterior Trunk	13	13	13	13	13
Left Buttock	2.5	2.5	2.5	2.5	2.5
Right Buttock	2.5	2.5	2.5	2.5	2.5
Genitalia	1	1	1	1	1
Left Upper Arm	4	4	4	4	4
Right Upper arm	4	4	4	4	4
Left Lower Arm	3	3	3	3	3
Right Lower Arm	3	3	3	3	3
Left Hand	2.5	2.5	2.5	2.5	2.5
Right Hand	2.5	2.5	2.5	2.5	2.5
Left Thigh	5.5	6.5	8.5	8.5	9.5
Right Thigh	5.5	6.5	8.5	8.5	9.5
Left Leg	5	5	5.5	6	7
Right Leg	5	5	5.5	6	7
Left Foot	3.5	3.5	3.5	3.5	3.5
Right Foot	3.5	3.5	3.5	3.5	3.5

the voltage and amperage of the current passing through the person's body as well as the resistance of the tissues to the current. The current will follow the path of least resistance and can destroy skin, blood vessels, muscle, or bone. It can also cause cardiac arrhythmias, electrolyte imbalances, and death.

Radiation burns have two sources: nuclear and solar (sun burns). Nuclear burns will not be discussed in this section.

BURN CLASSIFICATION

First degree burns involve only the epidermis. These burns appear dry, erythematous and often painful. They do not develop blisters and generally heal within 3 - 7 days without complication or scarring. These burns, when a small body surface area is affected, need local care only and analgesics. Very large burns (> 25% TBSA) of the elderly and infants require hospitalization.

Second degree burns extend into the dermis. Second degree burns are further classified as superficial partial-thickness and deep partial-thickness burns; depending upon the depth of dermal injury. Superficial partial-thickness burns affect the outer half of the dermis and are characterized by erythema, blanching to pressure, pain, and blister formation. Tissue beneath the blisters or exposed may appear mottled, weeping and moist. Healing occurs within 14 days and usually does not result in significant scarring. **Deep partial-thickness burns** involve the deeper half of the dermis and are sometimes difficult to differentiate from third degree, or full-thickness burns. Deep partial-thickness burns appear mottled, may be painful to touch, do not blanch with pressure, have blisters, and may be moist or dry. These burns require 3 - 4 weeks, or longer, to heal and are associated with significant scarring.

Third degree or full-thickness burns cause severe tissue damage to all layers of the skin, including the skin appendages (hair follicles, sweat glands), blood vessels, and nerve endings. These burns are pale white or charred, leathery or hard, dry, painless, insensitive to pinprick, and the skin does not blanch. Healing occurs over a protracted period of time after the need for skin grafting.

ESTIMATION OF BURN AREA

The severity of a burn is determined by calculating or estimating the extent of the burn injury with respect to the percent of the total body surface area (%TBSA). The **"rule of nines"** has been useful for determining critical, moderate, and minor burn injuries. The adult body is generally divided into surface areas of 9% or multiples of 9%, except for the genitalia (1%).

The "rule of nines" must be modified for children under 10 years of age because of the disproportionate size of the child's head and neck compared to the rest of the body. As the child grows, the "rule of nines" begins to approach the adult values. The Lund and Browder chart (Table 15.2) is more accurate for estimating the body percentages in both children and adults.

Another simple and convenient method of estimating the percentage of body surface area injured is to use the patient's own palmar surface; equivalent to 1 % TBSA.

BURN TREATMENT

First Degree Burns

- Cool compresses
- Aspirin or NSAID (unless allergic) for analgesia
- Skin emollients may be used to minimize dryness and soothe skin
- Follow-up with primary physician if needed

Second Degree Burn Treatment (less than 10% TBSA)

- Assessment of Airway, Breathing, Circulation, Disability, Exposure
- Remove all loose (nonadhering) clothing from burned area. Remove jewelry if burn is on an extremity.
- History, mechanism of injury including duration and type of exposure
- Examination for associated injury
- Burn estimation - % TBSA
- Fluid resuscitation and pain relief - NSAIDS to intravenous narcotics
- Administer anti-tetanus prophylaxis, if necessary.
- Application of sterile saline (not ice or water) compresses. Do not apply cold compresses to larger or deeper burns where a threat of hypothermia is possible.
- Leave small intact blisters alone. Sterilely debride ruptured blisters and devitalized tissue, particularly if blisters interfere with function (i.e., across joint surfaces).
- Gentle cleansing with normal saline, dilute povidone-iodine solution, or polaxamer 188 (Shur-clens).
- Drain and debride blister and devitalized tissue if blister is large or interferes with function (i.e., crosses the joint).
- Apply topical antibacterial cream (i.e., silver sulfadiazine) to burned areas except on facial burns and on patients with sulfa drug allergies or G-6-PD deficiency. Facial burns may be covered with polysporin or bacitracin ointment.
- Cover burned areas with a nonadhering, bulky dressing.
- Apply splint if burn crosses joints.
- Follow-up within 24 - 48 hours with primary physician, plastic surgery, burn center, or emergency department.
- Instruct patient to change dressings and cleanse burned areas every 12 hours followed by the application of the cream or ointment and sterile bulky dressing.

TREATMENT OF CHEMICAL BURNS

Immediate and copious irrigation with water, saline, or ringers lactate solution is required regardless of the type of chemical involved! Irrigation should continue for at least 30 minutes.

As mentioned earlier alkaline burns to the eyes are serious and must be irrigated immediately. Never attempt to neutralize an alkaline solution with an acidic solution, or vice versa, as more tissue damage will result from the release of heat (exothermic reaction).

The use of pH paper, if available, can be helpful to determine the type of substance involved and can be used to monitor the progress of irrigation (the end point is a pH of 7). However, DO NOT withhold irrigation to look for pH paper. The first priority is to irrigate the eyes.

Patients with tissue exposure to **hydrofluoric acid** (glass etchers, potters) require treatment before significant tissue damage results. The skin should be irrigated thoroughly and then an application of calcium gluconate or carbonate is placed of sterile gauze over the burn. Calcium deactivates the acid in superficial burns. A 32.5% slurry of calcium carbonate can be used for the treatment of hand and finger burns. Ten (10 grain) calcium carbonate tablets are ground into a fine powder and then combined with 20 ml of water-soluble lubricant gel (i.e., K-Y Jelly). The slurry is then massaged into the hand and fingers. About 10 ml of the slurry is placed in a surgical glove into which the affected hand is placed. Patients are instructed to move or massage the fingers / hand periodically and change the glove every 4 hours if pain persisted. (Chick, LR; Borah G, Plastic *Reconstiti Surg* 86:935-940,1990). A case series involving 9 patients, revealed that this method was effective in relieving pain in 8 out of 9 within 4-6 hours. The failure in the ninth patient occurred because the patient presented 24 hours after exposure.

Deeper hydrofluoric acid burns may require the slow, subcutaneous infiltration of 10% calcium gluconate solution into the burned area (dose equivalent to 0.5 ml per cm^2 of affected tissue). The administration of a local anesthetic prior to the calcium gluconate infiltration is recommended.

INHALATION BURNS

The physical signs of inhalation injury and airway compromise include:

1. Facial burns
2. Singed or loss of facial hair (eyebrows, eyelashes, nasal hairs, or mustaches)
3. Carbon deposits on the oropharynx and / or tongue
4. Carbonaceous sputum
5. Cough
6. Wheezing
7. Drooling
8. Hoarseness
9. Carboxyhemoglobin level > 15 %

BURN CENTER REFERRAL CRITERIA, after initial assessment and treatment at an emergency department, (may vary by locality):

- Partial thickness burns greater than 10% total body surface area in any age group
- Third degree in any age group.
- Second and third degree burns involving the hands, face, feet, or genitalia, perineum, or major joints.
- Any circumferential second or third degree burn involving the chest, extremities, neck, or digits
- Chemical and Inhalation injuries or burns
- Electrical burns, including lightning injury
- Burn patients with a significant pre-existing medical history (i.e., diabetes, immunosuppression, alcoholism, malignancy, and cardiac or pulmonary impairment).
- Any patients with burns and concomitant trauma in which the burn injury poses the greatest risk of morbidity or mortality. If trauma poses a greater immediate risk, then the patient may be initially stabilized in a trauma center before transfer to the burn center.

Principles of Primary Wound Management

TO ORDER ADDITIONAL COPIES OF:

Principles of Primary Wound Management -
A Guide to the Fundamentals

Visit and Order online at: **www.CliftonPublishing.com**

or

Complete the order form below and enclose payment (in U.S. Dollars) made
payable to:

CLIFTON PUBLISHING
6109 Fox Run
Fairfax, Virginia 22030-5949

Quantity

$16.00   Retail Price   _____

$14.00   Special Student and Resident Physician Price*   _____
           *for special discount price, please complete below
           School or Program Name _____
           Name of Dean / Program Director _____

                    Virginia residents add 4.5% sales tax $_____
                              TOTAL PURCHASE $_____

Payment method: Personal Check ☐ VISA ☐ MasterCard ☐

Credit Card Number _____

Card Expiration Date _____ (mm/yyyy)

Name of Card Holder: _____

Signature of Card Holder: _____

SHIPPING INFORMATION:

Name: _____

Address: _____

City: _____ State: _____ ZIP: _____

Telephone: (   ) _____
E-mail address **(used only to confirm credit card orders)**:

_____

Contact Clifton Publishing at:
E-mail: sales@CliftonPublishing.com
Telephone: (703) 502-3994   (9:00 a.m. - 6:00 p.m. ET, Monday-Friday)
FAX: (703) 502-1878 (24 hours)

About the Author

Mr. Mortiere is currently a practicing Physician Assistant in Emergency Medicine at the Inova Alexandria Hospital. He has more than 28 years of clinical experience in primary wound care in the emergency department setting. In addition to his present academic position, he has been an Adjunct Assistant Professor in Emergency Medicine at the George Washington University School of Medicine and Health Sciences (Washington, DC) and has been responsible for the instruction of medical students, resident physicians and physician assistant students during their emergency medicine wound management elective.

He has given numerous CME conferences and grand rounds lectures throughout the United States on wound management subjects over the last 20 years.